Praise for David Posen

Always Change a Losing Game
Now in its eighth printing and a national bestseller

"Everyone can relate to this book! Dr. Posen teaches us, through practical and entertaining stories, how to make our lives better in every way—and inspires us to take action!"
—Jack Canfield, co-author of *Chicken Soup for the Soul*

"This book makes change seem fun rather than a chore. Dr. Posen shows you how to turn dreams into reality. Begin reading any page—you'll not want to put this wonderful book down."
—Christine A. Padesky, Ph.D., co-author of *Mind Over Mood* and Director, Center for Cognitive Therapy, Newport Beach, CA

"For a change: a practical book full of the clinical wisdom of an experienced physician."
—Dr. Stanley E. Greben, Professor Emeritus of Psychiatry, University of Toronto

"This book is perceptive, instructive, productive and written in an entertaining fashion. It is a valuable addition to any growing person's library."
—Dr. Ron Taylor, Toronto Blue Jays team physician and former major league baseball player

Staying Afloat When the Water Gets Rough

"This book is an entertaining page-turner that empowers readers to manage change. Not only does Dr. Posen know what's going on here, he makes it easy for the rest of us to figure out."
—Peter G. Hanson, M.D., author of *The Joy of Stress* and *Stress for Success*

"David Posen has done it again! His survival guide for changing times is down to earth, reassuring and fun to read."
—Jack Canfield, co-author of *Chicken Soup for the Soul*

"David Posen is a very good advisor to anyone in transition. I recommend Staying Afloat When the Water Gets Rough *to anyone who's trying to make it through a bad stretch of white water."*
—William Bridges, author of *Transitions* and *Jobshift*

The Little Book of
STRESS RELIEF

The Little Book of
STRESS RELIEF

David Posen, MD

FIREFLY BOOKS

A FIREFLY BOOK

Published by Firefly Books Ltd. 2012

First printing

Publisher Cataloging-in-Publication Data (U.S.)
Posen, David B.
Little book of stress relief / David Posen.
2nd ed.
[208] p. : cm.
Includes index.
Summary: This resource is a helpful, inspiring and practical guide to alleviating the growing problem of stress in modern life.
ISBN-13: 978-1-77085-015-6 (pbk.)
1. Stress management. I. Title.
155.9/042 dc23   RA785.P6746   2012

Library and Archives Canada Cataloguing in Publication
Posen, David B.
The little book of stress relief / David Posen. -- 2nd ed.
Includes index.
ISBN-13: 978-1-77085-015-6
1. Stress management. 2. Stress (Psychology). I. Title.
RA785.P68 2012   155.9'042   C2011-906746-3

Published in the United States by
Firefly Books (U.S.) Inc.
P.O. Box 1338, Ellicott Station
Buffalo, New York 14205

Published in Canada by
Firefly Books Ltd.
66 Leek Crescent
Richmond Hill, Ontario L4B 1H1

Printed in Canada

The publisher gratefully acknowledges the financial support for our publishing program by the Government of Canada through the Canada Book Fund as administered by the Department of Canadian Heritage.

To my wonderful family, Susan, Jaime and Andrew,
who have enriched my life in ways I could never have imagined.

Contents

Acknowledgments

THIS BOOK HAD AN INTERESTING ORIGIN AND ODYSSEY. It was guided and shaped by many hands. Specifically, I would like to thank:

Paul Benedetti, my editor at Canoe—a mentor who became a friend—for teaching me how to write short columns, cheerleading my work and carefully reviewing my manuscript.

Dr. Greg Dubord, my colleague in cognitive therapy, who started my career at Canoe by recommending me to Paul Benedetti for the stress and lifestyle column.

Judy Love, my former assistant, who worked closely with me on the original Canoe columns—as typist and first-pass "editor"—who later critiqued this manuscript, and who always makes me laugh.

Beverley Slopen, my agent, advocate, coach and friend of many years, for her enthusiasm about this book.

Clare McKeon, my editor on this book, for her faith in me, her vision for this book, her guidance and her friendship.

Dr. Alan Brown, Dr. Robbie Campbell, Sue Hanna and Tony McLean, my esteemed colleagues and friends, for attentively reading yet another manuscript and giving honest and valuable feedback—most of which I acted on.

Judy Knapp, my former nurse, for her endless and ongoing support of all my books, for reading every word I've ever written and for being my auxiliary memory, remembering details of my writing better than I do.

Carol Anne McCarthy, my assistant, for organizing and easing my office life and for working with me on this book the past eight months. Her patience and tact with my multiple drafts has been exemplary.

Sue Sumeraj, my editor, who made the entire editorial process collaborative, collegial and fun. She has also promised to teach me a thing or two about shooting pool once this book has been put to bed.

Anna Porter and her team for their unflagging support, efficiency and professionalism, and for their warmth and kindness throughout our years of enjoyable association.

Lionel Koffler at Firefly Books for his interest, enthusiasm and support of this book.

Welcome

HAT IS THE ONE CONDITION every doctor shares with every patient? The answer is stress. It's everywhere. Whenever people find out I'm a stress consultant (from librarians in Toronto to limo drivers in New Jersey to techies in California), they invariably say, "Boy, could I use your services!" We all know about stress from experiencing it—even suffering from it at times. What we don't all know is what to do about it. That's what this book is about. I became interested in stress in 1981. Actually, "hooked" would be more accurate. I was a family doctor, and had just received a flyer advertising a seminar in Montreal on heart disease. The topics included nutrition, exercise, stress management and sexuality (that was probably the teaser—I guess someone figured that, even at a medical meeting, sex sells!). The conference looked intriguing, and a few days off appealed to me, so I signed up. Little did I realize, when I got off the train on that sunny June afternoon, that my work life was about to change forever.

The program featured three lectures on stress management. I was riveted. The presenter was a young, funny, self-admittedly nervous psychologist—and she was fabulous! Not only was the information fascinating, but I could see how helpful it would be for my patients. Even more compelling was the fact that I could see huge potential benefits for myself. I was not the most laid-back guy in the world. And working in a high-pressure job only added to my stress. Those first presentations explained things I had been experiencing all my life, but had never previously understood. I have pursued the subjects of stress theory and stress management with a passion that has not abated in more than 30 years.

Over time, I began to appreciate the widespread impact of stress on my patients—not only on their health and emotional well-being, but also on their energy, productivity, relationships, self-esteem and overall quality of life. I also made big progress in handling my own stress.

Evidence of stress surrounds us, from cover stories in magazines to newspaper tales of road rage; from people around us looking harried and hurried to the face looking back at us in the mirror.

Statistics bear this out. According to a 2010 *Globe and Mail* series on stress, Canadians experience an average of fourteen stressful episodes a week. Twenty percent of workers reported high levels of "crunch time when they feel over-whelmed by overcrowded inboxes and jammed weekly schedules." In 2008, close to two million Canadians were working more than fifty hours a week, up 23% from a decade earlier. Absentee rates for full-time employees increased by 21% in the past ten years. In the United States, the National Institute of Mental Health reports that more than 18% of adults suffer from an anxiety disorder each year. In his 2011 book *Nerve*, author Taylor Clark notes that "stress-related ailments cost the United States an estimated $300 billion per year in medical bills and lost productivity"–yes, *billion* with a "B." He states that, in the past ten years, anxiety has surpassed depression as the number one mental health issue in the United States. An online 2011 survey conducted by Harris Interactive on behalf of the American Psychological Association revealed that "more than one third (36%) of employees report they are typically stressed out during the workday" and "20% report that their average daily level of stress from work is an 8, 9 or 10 on a 10 point scale." Sort of catches your attention, doesn't it?

As if the news of current stress levels isn't bad enough, an earlier research study for the Heart and Stroke Foundation in 2000 showed that only 26% of Canadians felt that they knew how to handle their stress well. Dr. Rob Nolan, a Foundation spokes-man, said that people often cope with stress by engaging in harmful lifestyle habits. "About 75% of the respondents say their coping mechanisms include eating fatty comfort foods, watching TV, smoking cigarettes or drinking alcohol."

It seems safe to say that stress is a huge problem in our society and that most of us are not handling it very well.

We're living in stressful times: economic upheaval: debt crises in Europe; stock market gyrations and volatility; job shortages since the 2008 market meltdown; climate change; natural and weather-related disasters such as earthquakes and hurricanes; political instability and unrest; ongoing fear of international terror-ism and overall uncertainty. It's easy to feel overwhelmed and powerless. In the face of these enormous problems, one might ask how relevant it is to deal with the smaller issues of day-to-day life. Ironically, it may be *more* important in difficult times. I believe that the less control you have over your *external* environment, the more important it is to take control of your *internal* environment.

Aim to take control of the things you can control. These include the way you think, the way you behave and the lifestyle choices you make. If you manage these issues better, you'll have much more energy and resilience to deal with the larger, external forces that affect us all. And the good news is, you have more control than you think.

In the pages that follow, I will show you how to take more control of your life and handle stress with skill and confidence. I hope you find the journey both beneficial and enjoyable.

HOW TO USE THIS BOOK

Each chapter begins with a story or analogy, followed by relevant information and suggestions. The chapters end with prescriptions: specific, simple, concrete things you can do over the next week to put the ideas into action. My goal is to have the book serve as a guide for making gradual changes that will reduce your stress and improve your health.

The book can be read in three possible ways. You can read it straight through as with any other book. Or you can go directly to specific chapters that interest you. Or you can use it as an action-oriented manual, reading one chapter per week and implementing the prescription over the ensuing seven days. If you want to read about any subject in greater detail, there is a reading list at the end, organized by topic.

Whichever approach you take, I hope you find the book engaging, interesting, fun and of practical benefit as you deal with the stress of your life.

Is Stress a Friend or Foe?

A Lifesaver That's Also a Problem

YOU KNOW THE FEELING. You're driving along the highway minding your own business, listening to music and looking aimlessly at the scenery around you. Suddenly, in your rearview mirror, you see a police car coming up behind you, its red light flashing. You look down at the speedometer and realize that you're going well above the speed limit. Instantly, your heart starts pounding, your muscles tense, your hands squeeze the wheel, your breathing gets faster, your senses heighten and your mind becomes instantly alert (possibly calculating the fine awaiting you). Other silent changes occur as well: a rise in blood pressure, increase in blood sugar and fats, and so forth. Welcome to the world of stress reactions.

But then something unexpected happens. As you slow down, the cruiser catches up to you, pulls out into the passing lane and flies on by. You realize he wasn't chasing you after all. With a great sense of relief, you notice the stress reaction melt away over the next minute or two, and you slowly return to the relaxed state you were in before (well, almost).

We have all had experiences when our bodies go into a temporary state of "high alert." This is what the stress reaction was meant to do: turn on for short periods of time in situations of real or anticipated danger, and then turn off when the danger has passed.

Stress becomes a problem when there's too much, when it lasts too long or when it comes too often.

Unfortunately, in today's world, that is not what happens. Our stress reactions are activated far too often, and by situations that are not physically dangerous or life-threatening: rush-hour traffic, rude customers, being put on hold, computers that misbehave just when you're almost finished a document. We also react to ongoing situations: heavy workloads, deadlines, job insecurity, money worries and relationship problems. The result is that we switch on our stress reactions much more often, and for much longer periods of time, than nature intended. The resulting wear and tear on our bodies is not only unpleasant, but unhealthy.

We inherited the stress reaction from our caveman ancestors and, because of its protective nature, it was passed down genetically through the millennia (Darwinism in action). Think of a caveman confronting a wild animal or a warring tribesman, and you understand why the stress reaction was so vital to survival. In an instant, our forebear had to mobilize enough energy to either fight or run away from the threat to his physical safety. This is the classic "fight or flight response," mediated by adrenaline, cortisol and other stress hormones, which allowed our predecessor to either defend himself or flee.

"If it wasn't for stress, I'd have no energy at all!" Bumper sticker

We experience the same reaction today—and while it's crucial in a real crisis, it is inappropriate in our day-to-day lives. Not only are most of our stressors not life threatening, but fighting and running away are not exactly acceptable responses to most stressors. If someone is chasing you down a dark alley, the stress reaction can be lifesaving. But when the stress comes from an angry employer or a long line at the bank, it might be frowned upon to hit your boss or run down the street at high speed.

Dr. Hans Selye, one of the fathers of stress theory, defined stress as "the non-specific response of the body to any demand made upon it." The demand can be a threat, a challenge or any change that requires the body to adapt.

The first important thing to note is that the stress reaction lies in your *body*, not in the *situation*. Stress is not your child who won't go to bed, nor the person who just scooped your parking space. The stress reaction is what happens in your body *in response* to those situations.

Second, the stress reaction is neither good nor bad in itself. It depends on the circumstances. Stress is good when it protects us in times of danger or helps us to adapt to change. It is inevitable and necessary to survival. But it serves us in other ways, too, helping us study for exams or work toward a deadline. It's what athletes rely on to perform well in competition and what helps actors to give brilliant performances on stage. It motivates and stimulates us in our work, allowing us to be productive and creative.

Stress becomes a problem when there's too much, when it lasts too long or when it comes too often. That is when stress starts to create unpleasant symptoms and damage to the body. It's this negative or harmful stress that Dr. Selye called "distress."

> "Stress is like the tension on a violin string. You need enough tension so you can make music, but not so much that it snaps." Anonymous

So, is stress a friend or a foe? It can be either, depending on the situation. We need to learn how to decrease negative stress while still maintaining the positive effects. I call this balancing act "stress mastery," and we can all learn to do it better.

- Start noticing your stress reactions this week—even the mild ones.
- Note when they serve you well (high energy, focused concentration, excitement, etc.)
- Monitor when stress feels unpleasant or uncomfortable (tension, fatigue, lack of focus)
- Start to distinguish good stress from problem stress in your everyday life.

David Posen, M.D.

A police car in my rearview mirror still gets my attention. But I found the key to avoiding a stress reaction: I don't drive as fast!

Do You Know Your Signs of Stress?

How Does Stress Show Up for You?

PEOPLE OFTEN ASK, "How do I know when I'm having stress?" This reminds me of an old song title: "Am I in Love—or Is This Just Asthma?" Recognition of stress is important, because we can't deal with it if we don't know when it's happening. Other people are often aware of our stress before we are. They notice when we're brusque or abrupt; they see the tight jaw or fists that we don't recognize.

So what are the signs of stress to watch for?

Stress shows up in four ways: through physical, mental, emotional and behavioral symptoms.

1. PHYSICAL SYMPTOMS

In a classic stress reaction (the "fight or flight response"), the heart beats harder and faster (palpitations), muscles tense, breathing gets faster, the mouth goes dry. We may start sweating or feel a knot in the stomach. These are manifestations of acute stress.

Chronic stress shows up a bit differently. When I go through my checklist with patients, I start at the head and work down. I ask about headaches, dizziness, clenching the jaw or grinding the teeth, tight or sore muscles in the neck or across the tops of the shoulders, chest pains, abdominal symptoms such as indigestion, nausea, cramps, constipation or diarrhea. Back pain and tightness are very common. The hands and feet might tremble or feel cold or sweaty. As well, appetite may be lost or increased, and loss of interest in sex (decreased libido) is often reported.

> Fatigue is one of the most common symptoms of stress, but it is often overlooked or blamed on something else.

Fatigue is one of the most common symptoms of stress, but it is often overlooked or blamed on something else. Lots of people have trouble sleeping. There are three kinds of insomnia: trouble falling asleep, trouble staying asleep (frequent waking in the night) and early morning awakening (4:30 or 5:00 a.m.).

You've probably noticed that virtually all of these symptoms can be caused by other factors. Fatigue can result from diabetes or anemia; rapid heartbeat may reflect an overactive thyroid gland. You may need a doctor to help you decide if your symptoms are stress related or not. However, you can learn to look for patterns or groups of symptoms that usually indicate stress as the cause.

2. MENTAL SYMPTOMS

Do you have difficulty concentrating? That's a common stress symptom. I ask patients about problems with memory. Occasionally I hear: "What was the question again?" I inquire about trouble making decisions. One patient turned to his wife and said, "I don't know. Do I have trouble making decisions?" Your mind might race or go blank. One prominent politician's stress resulted in the loss of his usually terrific sense of humor.

3. EMOTIONAL SYMPTOMS

It's common for stressed people to feel nervous, anxious, tense, jittery, on edge, restless or agitated. They may feel irritable, frustrated, impatient or short-tempered. On the other hand, individuals may find themselves slowing down, feeling flat, apathetic, depressed, sad or blue.

4. BEHAVIORAL SYMPTOMS

When I was younger, I was a knee jiggler. It used to drive my sister crazy at the dinner table when I'd sit there with my knee rapidly bouncing up and down. Often she'd put her hand firmly on my knee to get me to stop. There were two fascinating parts to this: I was completely unaware I was doing it, and I could never move my knee that fast voluntarily. This habit results from excessive stress energy that the body tries to dissipate through muscular activity. Some people fidget or pace back and forth. Other behavioral symptoms include nail biting, compulsive eating, smoking, drinking, talking loudly, blaming or swearing.

"This guy was so tense he even had clenched hair." Unknown

Stress can manifest itself in dozens of ways. But most people have five or ten symptoms that are characteristic for them, their own galaxy of symptoms that they can learn to recognize. I get lower back pain but rarely get headaches. Others might get headaches, but never chest pains. Your pattern is usually the same each time, and you can learn to spot it. It might be a help if we sent out unmistakable signals when were experiencing stress: smoke coming out of our ears, hands going bright red or hair standing on end. However, if we learn to recognize our individual stress profile, we can become as good at detection as if there were steam coming out our ears. And identifying stress is the first step to doing something about it.

R̶x̶

- Today, take an inventory. Think about your symptoms when you feel stressed or upset. Write them down.
- Observe your body over the next few days whenever you're in stressful situations. Notice subtle signals you may not have observed before.
- Ask your family and close friends what they notice when you're stressed. What signs do they detect that you haven't noticed?
- Practice being more aware of these symptoms (without becoming too paranoid).

David Posen, M.D.

"Am I in Love—or Is This Just Asthma?" was one of those songs that are so bad they're good. Another of my favorite song titles is "How Can I Miss You If You Won't Go Away?"

Where Does Stress Come From?

The Sources Are All Around Us

ONSIDER THESE TWO SCENARIOS. In the first, I was in a room of our hospital emergency department with a patient who had become belligerent and had a menacing look on his face. Unfortunately, he was standing between me and the door, putting me in a captive position. Feeling threatened and in danger, I experienced an immediate stress reaction. Fortunately, I was able to calm him down while moving myself to the door.

Scenario number two: I was taking a taxi to the airport at 6:00 a.m., calmly relaxed and almost dozing off. Suddenly, I remembered something I'd forgotten to do the day before. Boom! A stress reaction as I realized my oversight and thought about the consequences. In both cases, the stress reactions were short, and one was much stronger than the other. But they were triggered by totally different situations: one an external threat, the other a spontaneous, internal thought.

What is comfortable to one person can be terrifying to another.

Once you're aware you're experiencing stress, the next question to ask is "Where's the stress coming from?" Dr. Hans Selye called these sources "stressors" or "triggers." Here's a helpful classification:

1. PHYSICAL OR ENVIRONMENTAL CAUSES

The first and foremost cause of stress is any physical threat to your safety. Beyond that, other physical stressors may include noise, big crowds or cluttered surroundings. I've had patients who walk the four flights of stairs to my office because they feel claustrophobic on the elevator. Some people experience stress in airplanes. Others find heights to be stressful. When I was nine, I climbed a 100-foot-high ranger tower. I was fine till the 75-foot mark when I made the fatal mistake of looking out over the forests below. Suddenly I was paralyzed with fear when I realized how high up I'd gotten. That was the last time

I climbed a 100-foot ranger tower! I also find it mildly stressful to work in rooms without windows.

Some people are bothered by certain circumstances, while others are not. Just as we get different stress symptoms, so also our stress is triggered by different situations, and what is comfortable to one person can be terrifying to another.

2. SOCIAL STRESSORS

Don't you just love it when people talk your ear off and won't let you get a word in edgewise? Or how about people who are rude and condescending and treat you like a speck of dust on their sleeve? One of the most common sources of stress is interaction with other people. This includes relationship problems, conflict with coworkers or bosses and feuds with neighbors. Certain people seem to cause you to feel stressed just by being around. Often it's a particular individual who appears to raise your stress level, but sometimes you react to general characteristics: people who are aggressive, critical, arrogant, loud, unreliable, negative or even boring. It's a wonder we get along as well as we do.

"Physics lesson: when a body is submerged in water, the phone rings." Unknown

3. INSTITUTIONAL STRESSORS

These are the rules and regulations of organizations or society at large. They include arbitrary restrictions, bureaucratic red tape, deadlines, expectations of immediate response (often because of technology), chains of command or pointless formalities. Office politics and endless meetings are high on this list.

4. MAJOR LIFE EVENTS

These are changes in life circumstances that can have a stressful impact for months or years, depending on the situation. At the top of this list is the death of a spouse, child or parent. But it also includes losing a job, moving to a new city, separation or divorce, and being a victim of crime or a serious car accident. Major life events can be stressful even when they're positive. In a fourteen-month period, I got married, bought a house, had a child (well, actually, my wife had the child) and changed careers—all good stuff, but still stressful.

In addition, effects from different events are cumulative. So losing a job and suffering a death in the family have a much greater impact than either of these by itself.

5. DAILY HASSLES

If you want to see a classic stress reaction, watch someone at the moment he realizes he's lost his keys or wallet. There's a look of shock on his face. He scurries around, retracing his steps, trying to find the lost item. The loss is hardly a major event, yet it can trigger a pretty impressive stress reaction. In the 1970s, psychologist Richard Lazarus coined the phrase "daily hassles" to describe relatively small or repeated situations in day-to-day living. Research showed that these were a better predictor of stress reactions and health problems than major life events. Examples of daily hassles include rising prices, home maintenance, having too much to do, fear of crime, driving in rush-hour traffic, repetitive house chores, parenting problems and health issues.

R x
- Grab a sheet of paper and take inventory. Write down the five categories and list the sources of stress in your life under each one.
- Monitor yourself throughout the week. Notice when you get upset and what triggers the stress. Add it to your list.
- Notice all the little irritants and hassles you deal with each day. Write them down.
- Pick one physical stressor you can change or eliminate and take action.
- Choose a social stressor and take one concrete step to minimize its impact on you.

David Posen, M.D.

These sources of stress are external. There's an even longer list of internal stressors!

Internal Sources of Stress
We Create Most of Our Own Stress

 MAN WAS TELLING ME about his problems at work. We devised a plan of action: he would discuss his grievances with his boss and ask for changes. It worked! His boss was receptive and supportive, and made changes to address his concerns. Problem solved, right? Well, not exactly.

One issue wasn't totally resolved—and that's what he chose to focus on. He also brooded over what had happened before and worried that the improvements wouldn't last. I gently reflected back to him that there was so much good news, so many positive signals, to be pleased about, and yet he continued to struggle and suffer. I suggested that he was actually making things harder for himself—and that the source of his stress was no longer the workplace situation, but the voice in his head.

If you ask folks where their stress comes from, most will identify external sources such as deadlines, noisy neighbors, sitting in traffic and telemarketers calling at suppertime. However, it may surprise you that the most common source of stress is ourselves. We create most of our own distress. When I share this thought with patients, I usually get one of two reactions. Most of them nod in agreement and say, "Yeah, I know. I'm my own worst enemy." But some take it as a blaming statement, saying in essence, "Oh, I see, not only am I feeling crummy, but now you're telling me it's all my fault. Thanks for the uplift!" I assure them that my comment is meant in a positive and constructive way. My premise is that if we create much of our own distress, then we can do something about it. We don't control other people's behavior, the weather or the economy. But we do have control over ourselves. So addressing our internal stressors is a logical starting point for reducing our overall stress.

We all have a little voice in our head that talks to us. (You may be relieved to

> We all have a little voice in our head that talks to us.

know you're not the only one hearing voices!) It's the voice that may be saying to you at this moment, "What's he talking about?" or "Oh, yeah, I know what you mean." Also called "self-talk" or an "internal tape," the voice comments on everything that goes on (like a combination editorial board/Greek chorus/cheering section/media critic). Some of its messages are positive: "This shirt looks really good on me" or "What a beautiful day. I can't wait to get outside." However, a lot of our self-statements have a negative tone. "Well, dummy, you blew *that* sales call" or "These people are really boring."

We react stressfully to certain situations through our internal conversations: "The service in this restaurant stinks" or "Who does he think he is, talking to me that way?" But we don't just react to real events, we also experience stress about what *might* happen, worrying about the stock market or an upcoming exam, for example. This is called "anticipatory stress." We even react to things that *don't* happen, such as not being invited to a party or someone not returning our phone calls. We can also get upset thinking about something that happened long ago, and trigger a stress reaction similar to the one that occurred at the time.

"Stress is a *fact* of life—but it needn't be a way of life." Unknown

Sometimes we feel stressed not because what happens is so bad, but because it was less than we expected. For example, a patient felt lousy after giving a speech. She told me, "My presentation went fine, but not nearly as well as I'd hoped. I counted on hitting a home run and only hit a double."

These are all examples of the little voice in our heads stirring up trouble. Talk about making life hard for ourselves! Add these internal conversations to things like drinking too much caffeine, overloading our schedules and getting into too much debt, and you start to see how many ways we can create stress for ourselves.

If this list seems daunting to you, don't be discouraged. First of all, realize that you're not alone. Second, recognize that awareness is the first important step to dealing with problems. And third, appreciate that, if we're the ones creating the stress, then we're in the best position to do something about it.

R̲x

• Start to notice each upset or stress reaction this week. Tune in to your inner voice and discern what it's saying. Write down some examples of your self-talk.

• Review the list and see if there's a pattern. Is the voice critical? Fearful? Complaining?

• Get feedback from family and close friends. Do they notice a pattern of negative comments from you?

• Look for other self-created stressors: Are you planning appointments too close together, so you feel rushed? Now that you have the Visa bill in hand, did you really need those new clothes? Write them down.

David Posen, M.D.

The good news about self-generated stress is we can fix it. We have more control than we think!

The Mind/Body Connection
Where Stress Really Comes From

T HE DETAILS ARE FUZZY, but it happened something like this: I was walking through a parking lot, when a car drove toward me. I expected it to stop, but instead it picked up speed. For an instant, I was paralyzed with fear. My heart was pounding, my whole body tensed up and my mind seemed to go blank for a few seconds. Just then, I recognized that the driver was a friend of mine and he was laughing. Realizing there was no danger, I laughed too—mostly with relief. This is a classic example of how our bodies react to situations that we judge to be dangerous. A stress reaction is instantly triggered to give us immediate energy to either fight or run away from the perceived threat.

This story illustrates an important—and surprising—point: Events and situations rarely cause stress (with obvious exceptions like being mugged on the street or your car going out of control). You can prove this premise in two ways. First, think of a situation that upset you on one occasion but not when it happened again a week later (for example, dawdling children or an unwanted knock on the door at suppertime). Second, think of a situation involving groups of people; you'll notice that not everyone reacts the same way. Take a flight delay at an airport. Some people get irate, others just shrug and go back to their reading and still others go up to the counter, get a voucher for the airport bar and walk away smiling. If the event or situation was causing stress, then everyone would be upset every time. Clearly, something else is going on here. Dr. Hans Selye summarized this phenomenon when he said, "It's not so much what happens to you that matters, but how you take it."

"It's not so much what happens to you that matters, but how you take it." Dr. Hans Selye

American psychologist Dr. Albert Ellis addressed this issue in a theory he called Rational Emotive Therapy (in *A Guide to Rational Living* by Albert Ellis and Robert A. Harper), to help us understand what happens between an event and

28

a stress reaction. I've summarized the theory in the following diagram, which I call "The Stress Pathway":

Stress Pathway

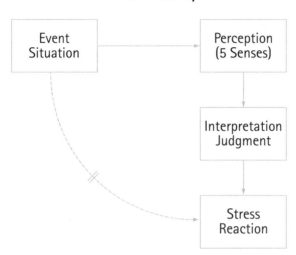

The Stress Pathway consists of four steps. First, an event or situation occurs, which we perceive through our five senses. We then immediately process the information intellectually, forming an interpretation or judgment about what happened. We give meaning to the event—which becomes our "reality." In the final step, our bodies respond to the interpretation with a stress reaction. This happens so fast that the situation itself appears to cause the stress reaction. But, if you tease it apart, you see these intermediate steps. We react not to the situation, but to our thoughts about the situation.

Here's an example. You're in a restaurant, waiting to meet a friend for a 1:00 lunch date. I happen along at 1:25. Your friend hasn't shown up yet. I notice you sitting alone and looking upset. I ask what's wrong, and you say, "Joe was supposed to meet me at 1:00, and he's not here." Curious to explore your stressful interpretations of this situation, I ask, "Why is that bothering you?" You probably want to say, "Duh, why do you *think* it's bothering me?" But instead you share the internal conversation you've been having with yourself: "It's rude to keep people waiting. I'm getting hungry. I have to leave at 2:00—now I'm going to have to wolf my food, and probably get indigestion. He doesn't think my time is important. He doesn't think *I'm* important. People should be on time. People who are late are inconsiderate. I feel like a jerk sitting here by myself. The waiter's getting upset because I'm tying up his table." Or, the stressful thoughts may relate to worry: "I'm afraid something happened to him. He may have been in an accident." Or the stress might result from self-doubt: "Maybe I got the arrangements confused. Maybe it wasn't today. Maybe I'm in the wrong restaurant."

"We see the world not as it is; we see the world as we are." Unknown

Let's return to the Stress Pathway. The objective situation is that Joe hasn't shown up yet. But your stress reaction is not a result of Joe's being late. It's a result of what you *think* about his being late (which is based on guessing and conjecture, not facts). You're interpreting his tardiness and reacting to those judgments.

Note: Not *all* self-talk is negative. After all, your own best companion is yourself! We make lots of positive self-statements that encourage and energize us. But it's the *negative* ones that cause the stress.

℞

- If you get upset about something this week, determine why you're upset. Tune in on the internal conversation you're having.
- Ask yourself, "Why is this situation upsetting me?" "Why is that a problem for me?" "What is it about this situation that's really bothering me?"
- Do this in writing—it's more powerful and gives you a record to refer back to.
- Notice whether your stress level is lowered after you understand why you got upset.

David Posen, M.D.

Analyzing your self-talk won't always reduce your stress. But understanding where your stress is coming from is an important first step in dealing with it.

By the way, the person who was late to meet you might have had a last-minute emergency at work, gotten stuck in traffic, been unable to find a parking spot—or he might have stopped off to buy you a gift and lost track of time!

Factors Influencing Our Stressful Interpretations

What's Your Inner Voice Saying?

O NE NIGHT, BACK IN 1987, our telephone rang at 1:30 a.m. Not exactly an earth-shattering event—but I reacted as if it was. Our bedroom phone was unplugged, so it took me a moment, waking from a deep sleep, to realize that the distant sound from the kitchen was a telephone ringing. Once I recognized what it was, my body went into a full-blown stress reaction. My heart was pounding, and I could barely get the jack into the wall because my hand was shaking. This reaction was quite out of character for me. I was a family doctor for seventeen years—my phone rang in the middle of the night all the time. I can't say I enjoyed it (there's an understatement), but I never had a stress reaction. However, the situation in 1987 was different. First of all, since I gave up general practice in 1985, our phone never rang after 11:00 p.m. But the second, more significant issue, was that a close relative was in the hospital. I immediately assumed something terrible had happened.

The main assessment we make is "Am I in danger or not?" If it's yes, our bodies react with a stress reaction. If we judge that we're not in harm's way, we usually relax.

As noted in the previous chapter, situations rarely, in themselves, cause stress in our bodies. They may *trigger* stress, but the real cause is the voice in our head that interprets and gives meaning to events as they occur.

Our interpretations don't take place in a vacuum. They're based on, or influenced by, a number of factors, including past experience and present circumstance or context. When my phone rang routinely after midnight, there was nothing stressful about it. But in the two years since I left general practice, a late-night phone call had become an unusual event. Because someone close to me was sick, my mind—and body—immediately jumped to conclusions.

Here's another illustration of the Stress Pathway (see page 29): How people react when a fire bell goes off. The event is a ringing sound that everyone hears. But not everyone reacts the same way. Some are blasé, while others think it's rather exciting. Some welcome the alarm as a break from work, while others get stressed or even panicky. Past experience strongly influences these responses. If the only fire alarms you've ever heard were false alarms or fire drills, you probably react casually. But two of my patients have told me they get very stressed when they hear a fire bell. In one case, the person's father was a firefighter; in the other, the patient had lost a close relative in a house fire.

Current circumstances also influence our interpretations. On several occasions, fire alarms went off while I was sitting in our hospital cafeteria. I was sitting on the main floor, beside a large window and very near an exit door. I assessed the situation and concluded I was perfectly safe—and continued to enjoy my lunch, as did all my tablemates. However, we reacted differently the day a fire engine arrived on the scene.

I also responded differently when I was on the ninth floor of a Toronto hotel and a fire alarm went off in the middle of the night. I didn't panic, but my wife and I took it seriously and moved quickly down the stairwells. Fortunately, the fire was nothing serious. But there is a funny sidebar to this story: when we hit the lobby, filled with sleepy guests and women in curlers, we noticed there were an awful lot of pets that had been slipped into rooms by patrons ignoring the "No Pets" rule, and a few very embarrassed people who were there not with their own spouses. Now, *those* people were certainly feeling stress!

"Reality is a collective hunch."
Lily Tomlin and Jane Wagner

So our stress reactions result not from what happens, but from our evaluation of what the event means. We take many things into account in reaching these conclusions—current conditions, similarity to past situations, beliefs, fears and expectations—and we do so very quickly. The main assessment we make is "Am I in danger or not?" If it's yes, our bodies react with a stress reaction. If we judge that we're not in harm's way, we usually relax.

There are two other significant evaluations: 1) feeling a lack of control (your computer glitches, for example, or there's a traffic tie-up when you're in a hurry) will usually generate some level of stress in your body; 2) anything that threatens your self-esteem (for example, when someone is angry at you or criticizes your behavior) will be experienced stressfully, if only briefly.

- The next time you have a stress reaction, large or small, step back and analyze your thoughts about the situation.
- Identify your self-talk. Ask "Why is this a problem for me? What's really upsetting me?"
- Then go a little deeper. Ask:
  — What from my past does this remind me of?
  — What fears, beliefs or insecurities may be operating here?
  — Is my self-image or self-esteem feeling threatened?
  — Am I feeling intimidated or rejected?

These insights are very helpful in understanding — and then defusing — stress reactions.

David Posen, M.D.

Incidentally, that 1:30 a.m. phone call was a wrong number. Ever since, I've trained myself to greet phones that ring in the middle of the night with "It's another wrong number" rather than "Oh my gosh, what's wrong?"

The Fascinating History
of Stress Theory

D R. HANS SELYE IS RECOGNIZED INTERNATIONALLY as one of the two fathers of stress theory (along with Dr. Walter Cannon). He was born in Vienna in 1907 and moved to Canada in 1932, where he worked at the University of Montreal.

Dr. Selye developed his concept of stress while studying medicine in Prague in the 1920s. He saw something that his classmates and teachers were missing. Much of medical education involved learning about different kinds of diseases and how to distinguish one from another by analyzing fine distinctions. (Oh, how I remember those days in med school.) A patient with pneumonia presented differently than a patient with tuberculosis; they both present differently than patients with heart failure or cancer. While everyone else was concentrating on the *differences* among these various diseases, Selye was struck by their *similarities*. His brilliance was in seeing what others couldn't see.

In 1926, as a second-year medical student on rounds, he noted that all the patients had a strikingly similar appearance: they were weak, tired, listless and apathetic, they often had muscle wasting and weight loss, and they even

> While everyone else was concentrating on the differences among these various diseases, Dr. Selye was struck by their similarities.

had similar facial expressions indicating that they were ill. He called this picture "the general syndrome of just being sick." His inquisitive mind started searching for the common elements affecting all of these patients. (His classmates were probably writing furiously, while he looked like he was daydreaming a lot.) This led him to identify the stress reaction as a cause of or contributing factor to most illness.

Selye's observations tied into the theories of Harvard physiologist Dr. Walter Cannon, who had earlier identified and named the "fight or flight response" (the body's response to feeling threatened or in danger.) But while Cannon saw the fight or flight syndrome as a positive mechanism used by the body to protect itself, Selye took it a step further. He realized that if the stress reaction goes on for too long, it causes damage to the body and leads to illness.

Another of Selye's unique and important findings was that the stress response in the body was the same no matter what the cause or source of stress (he called these sources "stressors"). His experiments on rats in 1936 showed that various stressors such as cold, heat, infection, trauma, hemorrhage, fear and the injection of noxious substances all produced the same effect. (Dr. Robert Sapolsky notes, in his wonderful book *Why Zebras Don't Get Ulcers*, that the rats had another stressor to contend with: Dr. Selye chasing them around the lab!) When the rats were later examined, they all had swollen and hyperactive adrenal glands, shrunken immune tissue (thymus gland and lymph nodes) and gastrointestinal ulcers. He had created an experimental model of "the syndrome of just being sick." He first called this reaction "a syndrome produced by various nocuous agents," but later, on noting that a wide assortment of stressors all produced the same response, named it the general adaptation syndrome (or G.A.S.)

> If the stress reaction goes on for too long, it causes damage to the body and leads to illness.

Selye's theory was that the body's supply of stress hormones eventually becomes exhausted, and this leads to illness. However, Sapolsky notes that new evidence demonstrates that these crucial hormones are not depleted. Instead, after prolonged exposure, it is the stress response itself that actually produces damage to the body.

So the good news is that our bodies are beautifully designed to protect us by mounting a stress reaction in response to various physical threats. The bad news is that the stress reaction cannot be sustained for too long. Eventually, the body suffers damage and either gets sick or dies. In other words, we benefit when our bodies go into a state of high alert to deal with a specific crisis, but we pay a price if the state of arousal goes on for too long. As so often happens, too much of a good thing becomes a problem. Fortunately, there's a lot

> "Stress is the spice of life. Without stress, life lacks excitement, challenge and a sense of adventure." Dr. Hans Selye

we can do to prevent the problems that result from chronic stress and deal with them more effectively.

Unrealistic Expectations
What Did You Expect?

WHEN WE DECIDED TO REDO our kitchen, we wondered what to do with the old cupboards. We were told about a broker who bought used cabinets and might pay us $500 to $600 for them. When he offered $900, it so exceeded our expectations that we accepted on the spot. To this day, I don't know whether we got a good deal. But it was much more than we expected, so we were happy.

Conversely, with a lot of our stress reactions, it's not the event itself that upsets us, but how it compares with our expectations. And when those expectations are unrealistic, we're almost guaranteed to feel some disappointment, frustration or even anger.

A woman was upset that her recently separated husband wasn't calling or seeing the children. I asked how much time he'd spent with the kids before the separation. "Not very much—that's another thing I'm angry about." I then asked why she expected him to show more interest in the children now than when he'd lived at home. She had no answer. I said: "I think your expectation is perfectly reasonable, but it's unrealistic given his track record over the years. I don't think it's going to happen. And the longer you expect this of him, the longer you'll stay upset." She agreed, and her anger slowly dissolved. Even though his behavior didn't please her, she reduced her stress by matching her expectation to the reality.

> "I strive for mediocrity—that way I always reach my goal."
> Bob Fuller

We all have expectations—of situations, of other people and of ourselves. But when they're unrealistic, they're like a trap we unwittingly set for ourselves.

UNREALISTIC EXPECTATIONS

1. About situations

Do you get upset every time your computer glitches? Do you get ticked off when the computer help line puts you on hold for ten minutes? How about when your car-phone signal breaks up or cuts out in tunnels or bad weather? How do you feel when your airline departure is delayed—again? These are some realities of life in the age of technology. My son, then twelve, understood this better than I did when I was getting frustrated with our computer: "Daddy, don't get upset. It's a new technology; they haven't worked out all the bugs yet." His expectations were realistic—mine weren't. Guess who had the stress?

2. About people

I once had a patient whose manager was driving him crazy. His boss, Roger, was generally uninvolved or nowhere to be seen. But when there was media coverage or they got an award, he was suddenly front and center to receive the kudos. My patient found Roger's behavior exasperating. Every week he told me another Roger story. One day I said, "Roger seems to be a model of consistency. I can see why you're irritated by his behavior, but why are you so surprised each time? Why are you expecting him to behave differently after all these years? Roger's just being himself." (A friend of mine calls this "Roger *doing* Roger.") I suggested he modify his expectations to conform with reality.

> His expectations were realistic—mine weren't. Guess who had the stress?

The next week he came in with another Roger story, but this time he was a little less upset: "Well, he did it again this week!" At the following visit, he said, "The guy never lets you down. Listen to this." By the third visit, he actually laughed as he told me another completely predictable story. As he slowly acknowledged the pattern, his stressful reactions diminished.

3. Of ourselves

People have a tough time if their expectations of themselves are so high that they can't be met. Perfectionists head this list. These people think they'll never make mistakes, they must always be right and they should never have a bad day.

The reality is that we can't do it all, we can't be all things to all people, we will make mistakes, we (including Serena Williams) won't win every game. And not everybody is going to like us, no matter what we do. It would be easier if we stopped putting such impossible expectations on ourselves.

Salespeople know they won't close every sale. In the insurance industry, there's a rule of thumb that ten cold calls yield three appointments, which result in one sale. That puts the hang-ups and rejections in perspective. It's all part of seeing things as they are, not as we'd ideally like them to be. One salesperson put it this way: "The law of averages says that rejections = sales!"

Rx

- Think of a situation that's bothering you right now (a quirky computer program, someone who's irritating you, a person who has let you down.)
- Try to articulate your *expectation* of this situation or person.
- Then look at the past record of similar situations or that person's behavior.
- Ask yourself: "Am I expecting too much?
- Adjust your expectations accordingly. Set your sights a little lower to reduce your stressful reaction to what's happening.

David Posen, M.D.

I wonder if we got a good deal on those cupboards after all. Oh well, the money was a bonus anyway!

Use Your Stress Reactions Wisely

You May Have a Finite Number

A PRIL 1993. BRIGHT SUN, warm temperature, a cloudless blue sky—a picture-perfect day for the first baseball game of the season. The Toronto Blue Jays had won the World Series six months earlier. Enthusiasm and optimism were at an all-time high. The game was sold out, but I had two tickets, twenty rows up from first base. I was taking a friend visiting from Baltimore. How convenient—the Jays were playing the Baltimore Orioles. And it was a day off from work. All in all, a great setup for a relaxing and stress-free day.

We set out early for the SkyDome, and got there in good time. All we had to do was park the car. That's when I realized that thousands of my fellow fans had also arrived early. We started driving around to find a spot, but traffic was gridlocked and time was ticking along. As we got close to game time, I thought about abandoning my car or giving it to a pedestrian—anything to get rid of it! There really is something to be said for public transportation.

Through this entire exercise in futility and frustration, I noticed my stress level rising. That amused me for two reasons: 1) this was only a baseball game; and 2) I'm ... er, uh ... a stress doctor.

It reminded me of a fascinating three-part concept I once read regarding our capacity to deal with stress. First, what if our bodies were programmed to withstand or experience a set number of stress reactions over our lifetime, and when we exceeded that number, our bodies would be overwhelmed and pack it in and we would die? The idea has a certain logic to it. Think of a car motor. After a certain number of piston thrusts, motors just wear out. It's not all that big a leap to think that our bodies have a finite capacity as well—after so many heartbeats, so much wear and tear, our time would be up. The second part of the theory is that each of us has a different capacity to withstand repeated stress—a set number of stress reactions

> "We can choose what stresses us, and for how long." Dr. Hans Selye

programmed into our bodies. My number might be 281,000, yours might be 308,000, and so on. Finally, although we each have a finite number of stress reactions programmed into us, none of us knows our own quota.

If we accept this theory, it would be smart to ask ourselves which situations warrant the expenditure of one of our precious stress reactions. Say the movie you're going to is sold out. Is that worth using up one of your stress reactions? If your preschooler spills his juice, does that warrant a stress reaction? The world starts to look different if we can *choose* what we allow to upset us. And that is exactly what we *can* do!

Not only can we choose what stresses us, we can also choose how long to hold on to our stress. A very upset patient came to see me. Four hours earlier, she'd been waiting to use a pump at a gas station. When the previous car finally pulled out, another car darted in from nowhere and took the pump before she could move forward. She got out of her car, asserted herself, even argued with this interloper. All to no avail. She was incensed. Several hours later, she was still in a state of agitation. This was not serving her well. It was an example of the price we pay when we hold on to stress longer than necessary.

R_x

- For the next week, notice what type of situations trigger your stress. Keep a log.
- Start to ask yourself, "Is this situation worth using up one of my stress reactions?"
- If you decide it's not worth it, choose to let it go. Don't rise to the bait.
- If you do get upset, ask yourself, "How much stress does this situation warrant? How many minutes do I want to stay upset about this?"
- Continue to practice staying calm, especially when it comes to the little things. Notice how easily you can take control of the extent and duration of your stress reactions.

David Posen, M.D.

Incidentally, we got to our seats after the first inning and had a great afternoon— unlike a guy in our row who arrived in the third inning and fumed for the next hour. I wonder how many stress reactions he used up that day.

The Work–Life Balancing Act

It's Time to Reverse the Trend

H ANG AROUND THE WATER COOLER in any workplace, and you'll notice one of two things: either no one's there because no one has time to hang around anymore, or the people you see are all talking about how they don't have time to be standing there. Everyone's got too much to do and not enough time to do it.

Issues bubble to the top of the stress agenda from time to time. In the mid-late 90's it was dealing with rapid change. In the past 10-12 years, it's been work–life balance. In fact, that's the seminar topic most requested of me for the past decade.

In October, 2011, The Canadian Index of Wellbeing report was released after a 12-year study. It measured how people were faring in their day to day lives based on 64 indicators in eight areas such as living standards, health, leisure, culture and how we spend our time. They found that Canada's GDP rose 31% between 1994 and 2008, while the Index of Wellbeing increased by only 11%. According to the *Toronto Star*, "the time crunch and income inequality both went in the wrong direction. We're spending more time working and less time visiting elderly parents or playing with our kids." Roy Romano, Chair of the Index advisory board, said most Canadians are "running so fast and basically standing still that we do not have the opportunity to enjoy things that really matter in life."

The goal is balance. But the key is permission.

In the United States it's no better—or worse. A 2010 study by the National Sleep Foundation showed that the average worker spends nine hours a day at the workplace topped off by another several hours at home—decreasing total sleep time during the week. How did we get ourselves into this tangle? And more important, what can we do about it?

It would help to learn a new vocabulary relating to work–life balance. At the top of that list I'd put the word "permission." I used to think the word "leisure" meant rest and relaxation until I looked it up in the dictionary. I was surprised to find that it comes from the Latin root *licere* (the same root as the word "license"), and it literally means "permission." Anything you do out of freedom and choice is a leisure activity, even hiking or playing squash. Leisure doesn't have to be sedentary. It just has to be something that you choose to do. We're short on leisure not because there isn't enough time, but because we don't allow ourselves to *make* or *take* the time.

One of the best parts of my job is giving people permission to take time for themselves. A patient was working six days a week and spending the seventh day at home with his family. But he missed playing golf. He had given up golf because he felt he should spend his only free day, Sunday, with his wife and children. While I respected his values, I suggested that he could play a round of golf and still have twelve hours to spend with his family. He felt uncomfortable with the idea. Finally I said to him, "I'm giving you permission to play golf this Sunday. Just see what happens. Tell your family that it's my idea. Let's just do it as an experiment." He agreed to give it a try.

> I wrote him a prescription for "1 game of golf this Sunday." Then he asked for a second script—for a trip to the Bahamas!

At his next visit, he reported that he'd played golf and enjoyed himself. He even thanked me for giving him permission. But he also got some interesting feedback from his family. They noted that he was more relaxed, in a better mood, and more involved with them than he had been on other Sundays. They said he had previously been preoccupied, withdrawn, irritable, restless.

The pleasant surprise from this experiment was that his family benefited from his recreational time, because he was more fun to be around when he had done something for himself. The following week he gave *himself* permission to play. What he had seen as a zero-sum game (if he won, his family lost), turned out to be a win-win situation: he still spent the majority of the day with his family, but in a better mood and frame of mind.

The key to this story is balance. By making time for a leisure activity, he met his own needs *and* those of his family. His decision wasn't "me first" or "me only," but "me too."

• Step back and look at your life. Do this quick survey to see where you stand:

1. On a scale of 1 to 10, rate your current **work–life balance**.

1	2	3	4	5	6	7	8	9	10
Awful								Utopian	
(all work)								(perfect balance)	

2. On a scale of 1 to 10, rate your current **stress level**.

1	2	3	4	5	6	7	8	9	10
Minimal							Off the wall		
(blissed out)							(burned out)		

• If your balance is low and stress is high, pick one activity you'd like to be doing but have neglected (reading, playing golf or tennis, taking a hot bath, playing the piano, having lunch with a friend, getting a massage).

• Make plans to do that activity at least once in the next week.

• If you feel uncomfortable, tell yourself "I'm giving myself permission to do this. It'll be fun, and balance is important."

• If you're still faltering, seek out someone who will give you permission to get you started.

• Make plans to do it again (or something different) next week.

David Posen, M.D.

Do something for yourself every day. And do it without guilt. The goal is balance. But the key is *permission*.

The Power of Permission

Listen to Your Instincts

A WOMAN APPROACHED ME after one of my seminars. She was struggling with a time management problem, trying to juggle several elements of her life. In addition to a full-time job and raising two preschool children, she was spending fifteen hours a week on starting a new business with a friend. Having difficulty doing everything, she'd called a radio talk show to explain her dilemma to a guest expert. His response was, "Well, you're just not organized," and he gave several suggestions about being more efficient. She'd already been feeling overwhelmed, but after hearing from the expert, she also felt guilty for being unable to manage.

I asked her two questions: "What do you really want to do?" and "What do you think you could comfortably handle?" She said she couldn't keep doing it all. I told her "It's tough to work fifty-five hours a week and still have anything left for your family and yourself. When your kids are older, maybe you can rethink the situation. But for now, it sounds like a full-time job and raising two children is quite enough. Maybe your friend can find someone else to partner with." The sense of relief that radiated from her was almost palpable. She thanked me for validating her feelings and for supporting what she really wanted to do.

> Too many people give up parts of their lives to meet other people's goals.

What is this story about? Why did she need advice from "experts" when she already knew what was right for her? I think she was looking for *permission*. She wanted an authority figure to sanction her decision, to tell her it was okay to scale back. Perhaps she was also seeking external support to justify her decision to her friend.

We often need someone's approval to give us courage to act. One of my patients came to see me because she had to make a big decision and wasn't sure what she should do. It involved cutting back her work hours so she'd be able to spend more time with her small children. She was reluctant to even inquire about the possibility because "I'll look unprofessional. It's a risk—what if they look unkindly on it?" She worried about the implications for her career if she appeared to be less dedicated to her work.

In exploring the pros and cons to help her make this decision, it struck me that she was actually quite clear about what she wanted to do. I told her, "You don't sound like someone struggling with a tough decision. It seems to me that you've made up your mind. But you're stuck at the stage of acting on the decision."

She replied, "You're right. But I just needed your permission."

In truth, she really needed permission from herself. But she didn't realize that until we were into the conversation. What she viewed (and presented to me) as a problem of indecision was really an issue of inaction. And the key to moving forward was not making a choice but giving herself permission to implement that choice.

This story illustrates that we sometimes need an external voice to affirm our behavior or to reinforce our desire to do something. Permission is a form of endorsement from other people. We need someone to give a blessing to a course of action that, in our heart of hearts, we want to follow, but somehow cannot allow ourselves to pursue.

Ultimately, we need to get past our reliance on other people. If we're to achieve the lives we envision, we need to get better at giving ourselves permission to choose what feels right and then act on it. This is not about acting selfishly—it's about self-determination and self-reliance. It's about living according to our own values and priorities, not somebody else's. Too many people give up parts of their lives to meet other people's goals.

> Ultimately, the person you need permission from is yourself.

Whether you're making a career change or plans for the weekend, start listening to your inner voice and let it guide you. Giving yourself permission is one way to take more control of your life.

- Identify one thing that you want to do (or stop doing), but haven't been able to act on.
- Ask yourself why you're stuck. Do you not want it badly enough? Do you think you'll feel guilty if you do it? Are you concerned about what others might say?
- Ask yourself whose permission you need to help you move forward.
- If you need someone else's permission, discuss it with him or her and ask for support.
- If it's your own permission that's required, grant it to yourself on a trial basis—"I give myself permission to do this for a week/month/year/semester as an experiment." Then evaluate the decision (and its benefits or downsides) as you go along.

David Posen, M.D.

Giving yourself permission to make changes or to do things differently is a liberating experience. And it gets easier the more you do it!

Where's the Pressure Coming From?

Look Around You. Then Look in the Mirror!

I T STARTED OUT AS A CONVERSATION about constipation. (Stay with me here—I don't plan to go into graphic detail.) My patient was an attractive young woman who had been a conscientious student and was now out in the business world. She came to me with abdominal complaints, so I asked about her eating habits. It surprised me to learn that she wasn't eating lunch. I thought, "What kind of employer makes people work through their lunch hour?" But, when I asked, she admitted this was not company policy. The pressure was coming from her. She felt that skipping lunch was the only way to get her work done.

> Type-A perfectionists push relentlessly for both quantity and quality—they're always fun to watch!

Overwork is often more complicated than a demanding boss and a compliant employee. Let's look at some sources of workplace pressure that cause people to work long hours and upset their work-life balance. Incidentally, these factors also lead to overload in the *non*-work part of our lives.

1. **External demands:** These come from bosses and clients, coworkers and customers. They involve not only what people want you to do, but also the standard of excellence they expect from your efforts.

2. **Deadlines:** It's not enough that people ask you to do stuff, but they toss in a time limit while they're at it. You feel a lot more squeezed if they need it by Tuesday morning than if they want it by Thanksgiving.

3. **Peer pressure and corporate culture:** These include anything from a raised eyebrow when you leave early to a sarcastic comment if you go out for a walk on your lunch hour. From the example set by executives who come in on weekends to someone saying, "We don't do that around here" when you make

a personal phone call. The messages, whether stated or implied, exert gentle pressure to conform.

4. **Internal demands:** These are our own expectations and standards. Type-A individuals are always trying to do more, while perfectionists have very high standards of excellence. (Type-A perfectionists push relentlessly for both quantity *and* quality—they're always fun to watch!)

5. **Perception of danger:** "If I'm late with this project, my boss will kill me." "If I don't come in this weekend, it could affect my performance appraisal." We give ourselves internal messages about the negative consequences that will result if we don't get things done. This cranks up the pressure meter.

6. **Evaluation of our ability to accomplish tasks:** Pressure is affected by our level of confidence. If I look at a mountain of work and think, "There's no way I can possibly get all this done," I will feel a lot more anxious than if I say to myself, "Boy, there's a lot of work here, but I know I can handle it."

There are some important points to note about these six sources of pressure:

- The first three are external, but the second three are internal. We often think of pressure as being exerted from outside us, but we bring a lot of it on ourselves.

- We don't control the first three factors, but the last three are all under our direction.

- Even though we don't *control* the first three items, we can *influence* them. For example, we can decline requests from others under certain circumstances. We can negotiate deadlines if they're too tight or unrealistic. We can check to see if our perceptions about corporate culture are accurate. (I had a patient who thought bringing her child to work was unacceptable. Then one day she had no choice—and she was pleasantly surprised to get no flak. In fact,

> "The harder you push yourself, the harder your self pushes back." Anonymous

people were playing with the kid all day!) And we can gently challenge or push back against peer pressure when necessary.

> **Rx**
>
> - Acknowledge that you can't do everything asked of you. Stop trying!
> - Look at your schedule today. Set realistic time frames for the completion of each item.
> - Protect your time. If your day is already full, say no to new requests, or schedule them for another day.
> - Start to monitor your internal messages of doom. Notice how often you scare yourself with negative self-talk.
> - Refute your negative messages. The sky isn't going to fall if something is delayed or done less than brilliantly.
> - Find one thing to let go of this week or to do less than perfectly.
>
> You have more control than you think. Start using it.
>
> David Posen, M.D.

So what happened to my patient who was working through her lunch hour? She began to go out for lunch, and quickly found that the relaxation was just as important as the food. And she admitted that the "boss" who'd been pushing her was her. Oh yes, one more outcome: her constipation did improve.

Peer Pressure and Corporate Culture
It's Time to Speak Up

A PATIENT TOLD ME about his unrelenting stress at work. When I suggested he take some breaks to get out of the pressure cooker, he explained how difficult that was. The office was in a sub-basement, far from the street-level doors, so even getting some fresh air took too long. "What about lunch?" I asked. He replied, "I can't get out for lunch. They don't take lunch." Someone actually told him, "We don't do that here." Feeling like a mole, he ignored this directive and went out at lunchtime. But not for long. His coworkers showered him with snide remarks until he adopted their workaholic tendencies.

In a hundred different guises, peer pressure and corporate culture have a huge impact on employees. They are also major factors affecting work–life balance.

Every organization has a personality. Some are stodgy, others fun. They might be aggressive or laid back, secretive or open, risk averse or innovative. Corporate culture can be constructive, positive and a source of pride. Or it can be a problem, meaning long hours, weekend work, self-sacrifice or neglecting your family.

One of my patients pulled the odd all-nighter at the office. When I asked him who else was around in the middle of the night, he said, "More people than you would believe." Some companies set up meetings on Sunday mornings and view attendance as a litmus test of commitment and loyalty. These customs are all examples of "This is the way we do things here."

Peer pressure is less institutionalized. It's the way individuals or groups try to influence the behavior and attitudes of others. Sometimes peer pressure may reflect the corporate culture, sometimes not. Managers and supervisors are the gatekeepers of company

> In many companies, the important messages are unspoken—and actions still speak louder than words.

policy on work–life balance. They can support or sabotage the official plan. Employees who want to leave early (for a parent's medical appointment or a child's soccer game) don't call the CEO to ask for permission. They clear it with their supervisor—and that person's attitude will determine the outcome. While corporate culture develops over time, peer pressure is usually exerted by forceful personalities and/or entrenched personnel. For better or worse, they're the ones with the power. They are often workaholics or Type-A people, highly driven individuals who in turn drive other people hard.

How people act as they move up the hierarchy is important. When people have experienced unpleasant systems or felt exploited, they usually adopt one of two attitudes: 1) "I was treated badly and, when I get some power, I'm going to do the same thing to the people below me," or 2) "I was treated badly, and I will never do this to anyone else."

Often there's a difference between stated policy and what people (especially executives) actually do. More companies are espousing the work–life balance message, but senior people are still coming in early, leaving late, and registering subtle disapproval when others don't do the same. In many companies, the important messages are unspoken, and no matter what the policy says, actions still speak louder than words.

The most strategic way to challenge peer pressure and change corporate culture is to build consensus. Don't take on the system alone. Talk with others and see who agrees with you. Develop a group to lobby for change. Then present your ideas together. In the mid-70s I stood up at one of our Department of Family Medicine meetings to speak against the sale of cigarettes in our hospital. After one or two lukewarm comments, the issue was dropped. A senior colleague gave me some good advice as we walked out: "That was a good idea, but you should plan more carefully when you raise something like that. It would've been better to gather support ahead of time, and to have some people speak in favor of the idea. If you'd been better organized, you might have convinced more people."

> Challenging the status quo is not about rebellion or mutiny—it's about trying to improve the workplace environment and experience.

Other thoughts on promoting change:

- **Don't assume that the corporate culture is unchangeable.** You can influence company practices. If you're a new hire, you can bring fresh ideas to the organization. If you're a veteran, you have added influence based on seniority—an opportunity (and responsibility) to shape and move the corporate culture in positive directions.

- **Dare to be different. Have the courage of your convictions.** Introduce some humor into a stodgy company or meetings that get too serious. Organize a group to play Frisbee at lunchtime or to go for an afternoon walk.

- **Support initiatives proposed by others.** Get behind other colleagues when you agree with their ideas.

- **Bide your time.** If you're new on the job, take time to observe the corporate climate and your new colleagues. Don't flaunt the unwritten rules on day one. But don't compromise your principles either. In some areas (taking lunch, leaving on time) establish your own style from the outset—and show that you can pace yourself and *still* do good work.

- **Finally, you may decide it's necessary to leave.** If you feel the company's values and practices are unacceptable to you, you may need to find a more compatible job.

Rx

- Ask yourself, "What is one thing I'd like to see changed in my workplace?"
- Ask people "Why are we doing this" or "Why is this done in this way?"
- Start to build consensus, and lobby for change in a constructive (not rebellious) way.
- Take one action on your own. Don't announce what you're doing. Others may follow your lead.
- Identify one person who is pressuring you and ask to discuss the situation.

David Posen, M.D.

Anyone can affect corporate culture. It's not changed only from the top down. If you work in a company, you are, by definition, part of the culture. You're a stakeholder. You have just as much right to help shape the culture as anyone else in the organization. It's time to speak up!

Setting Boundaries and Limits
Enough Is Enough

PINBALL MACHINES HAVE A TERRIFIC WAY of demanding respect: if players push them around too much, they go "tilt" and shut down. No second chances. That's a pretty impressive way of setting limits on the amount of abuse they're willing to take. When it comes to work–life balance, we too need to set limits to protect ourselves. We could use the word "tilt," but I have another suggestion.

When I was in general practice and reached a critical mass of office patients, phone messages and paperwork, the word "Enough" would flash through my mind like a big neon sign. I'd stop, sit down with my nurse and start delegating like crazy—finally making decisions I had been putting off for days. The pile of charts on my desk would fade within minutes, leaving me with a manageable workload and a great sense of relief.

"Enough" is another word to add to our work–life balance vocabulary. The work day is getting longer and faster, and it's open-ended. To get some control of this situation, we need to start asking, "How much is enough?" How much is enough work time? How much is enough success? How much is enough money?

Let me share three stories. A friend of mine was lamenting his heavy workload. A self-employed professional, he was inundated with clients, paper, phone calls and e-mails, surrounded by files and plagued by constant deadlines. His work routinely spilled over into his evenings and weekends. He said he had no choice because he had so much to do. I asked, "What do you mean you have no choice? Why did you take on so many clients in the first place?" He said, "Hmm, I see what you mean. I guess I did have a choice."

> Working longer or harder is not only unproductive, it's counterproductive.

A patient recounted a whirlwind trip to Chicago to finalize a business deal. He put in several eighteen-hour days with a large team of lawyers, accountants and business people before finally dragging himself home in a state of exhaustion.

I asked, "What was the compelling urgency that had all these people working crazy hours to complete this transaction?" He said, "That's just the way they do business there." Then he added, "Do you want to know the worst of it? After I left, they were already revving up for another marathon session to close the next deal. For them, it never stops." Yikes!

The third story involves a person who got home for dinner only twice a week. In addition to his full-time job, he volunteered his time to five community organizations! A nicer guy you couldn't find, but he was pulling himself in so many directions that he barely had time for his family.

I asked each of these people two questions: "Why are you doing this?" and "How much is enough?"

Too many of us are on overload. People who work long hours are fooling themselves. Very few folks can put in more than ten hours a day (or fifty hours a week) and still be productive. After that, everything takes longer because we become tired and inefficient.

This is illustrated by the classic Yerkes-Dodson Law, which shows the relationship between performance and stress.

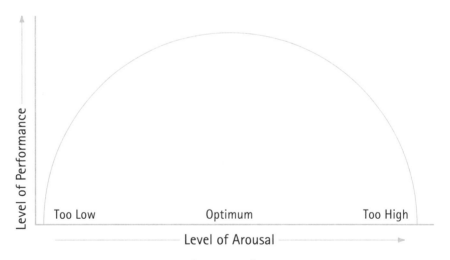

Relationship between arousal (and stress) and performance according to the Inverted-U Hypothesis and the Yerkes-Dodson Law

In the first part of the curve, motivation or stress actually improves our efficiency. But past a certain point, the reverse occurs: ongoing stress impairs our effectiveness. In fact, working longer or harder beyond that point is not only unproductive, it's counterproductive—it just prolongs the distress and inefficiency.

> "People who spend most of their time putting out fires are usually also the arsonists."
> Dan Sullivan

Instead of pedaling harder and faster, we should be pulling back for some recovery time. Better yet, we should avoid the downside of the curve altogether. In other words, we need to pace ourselves. This is where setting boundaries and limits is so important.

Here are some parameters I've adopted to maintain efficiency in my work and balance in my life:

- I work from 8:00 a.m. to 6:00 p.m., with time for lunch and an exercise break in the afternoon.

- I work only a few evenings a month.

- I rarely work on weekends.

- I almost never travel for business on Saturday or Sunday.

- I rarely go out more than two evenings in a row, even socially or to play sports.

- I rarely check e-mail in evenings or on weekends.

These are boundaries I've established over the years. They're not hard and fast, but I don't violate them very often.

One can also establish boundaries by location. For example:

- Don't work at home.

- If you do work at home, limit yourself to only one room or place in the house.

- Don't work on vacation—no laptop, smartphone or work-related reading.

- Look at your schedule. Do you have a routine for work hours? Are you satisfied with your starting and finishing times?
- Decide what time you want your work day to begin and end.
- Pick one realistic change you can make in the next week (leave for work thirty minutes later or go home an hour earlier at the end of the day). Evaluate after one week.
- Choose one "bad habit" you've picked up (checking your e-mail before you go to bed, calling in for messages on Saturday morning), and commit to changing it.

David Posen, M.D.

Establish limits. Ask yourself "How much is enough?" and set boundaries accordingly. Then say "Enough" before your body says "Tilt."

Saying No
Being Selective Is Self-Protective

WHEN MY OLDER SON WAS TWO, there were times when I told him to do something and he simply said "No." I'd look at him in amazement, admiring his courage and amused by his determination. I'd say to my wife, "Doesn't he realize that I'm 6'1" and he's only 3 feet tall? Would I say that to a twelve-foot giant?" And yet there he was, standing his ground!

There's an irony here: small children have less trouble saying No than adults do. This cheeky little kid had a skill that most grownups struggle with. I ask people in my seminars how many of them are able to say No in appropriate circumstances, and do so with comfort and confidence. Very few hands go up. A self-employed professional who was overwhelmed by work told me he had trouble saying No to his clients. When I asked him why, he said sheepishly, "Because they won't like me."

A second irony is that one of the most empowering words in the English language is also one of the shortest. When people can't say No, they get overloaded, stressed and resentful. People who are able to say No have less pressure and feel more in control of their lives. They also have more free time, increased energy and feel better about themselves. Pretty big payoffs from such a small word.

Learning to say No does not mean we become difficult or uncooperative. After all, collaboration and teamwork are essential in today's workplace. Saying No is about self-protection. It acknowledges that we can't do everything nor keep everybody happy, and

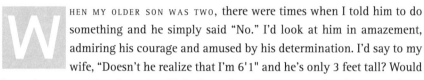

If you do it properly, you never actually use the word "no."

we drain ourselves if we try. Saying No is about recognizing our limits and being selective in what we choose to do.

WHEN TO SAY NO

No does not have to become your favorite word, or the first thing you say after "Hello." Nor do you have to say it often. Even used 5% of the time, it will serve you well.

When is it okay, appropriate—even necessary—to say No? This is a permission-giving exercise. Most of us have no difficulty saying No if we have to leave work early to catch a plane. Here are some other situations when it's okay to say No:

1. When you're exhausted or stressed out.

2. When you're overloaded and out of time.

3. When you have higher, more pressing priorities.

4. When it's not your job or responsibility.

5. When it's not your area of expertise and someone else could do it better.

HOW TO SAY NO

The next question is how to say No in a way that reasonable people will accept. Here's a third irony: if you do it properly, you never actually use the word "no."

1. **Express your wish to help:** "I'd like to do that for you" or "I wish I could be helpful."

2. **Give an explanation:** "I'm working on a tight deadline" or "I have to get to a dental appointment." You don't have to get highly personal.

3. **Offer an alternative:** "Barb's really good at this, and she loves to do it" or "I won't be able to do it, but I can show you how to do it."

4. **Offer to do it later:** "I can't help you now, but I can do it next Tuesday."

5. **Offer to do part of the task:** "I won't be able to do all of it, but I'd be happy to do this part for you."

6. **Ask her to help you prioritize:** "Which of these projects would you like me to set aside in order to do this one?" She'll likely say one of two things:

a) "I didn't realize you had that much on the go. I'll deal with this another way."

b) "Set that one aside and do this instead."

Either way, she accepts ownership of the decision. She can't come back to you next week and say, "Where's the such and such report?" when she's the one who told you to put it away.

> "Things that matter most must never be at the mercy of things that matter least."
> Goethe

7. **Ask for time to think about it:** "Can I get back to you in an hour? I'll try to rearrange my schedule."

    Then, if you can't fit it in, call back and say, "I'm sorry, it's not going to work. Perhaps another time."

8. **Ask what it's for:** Help her clarify her situation and real needs.

Saying No is an important life skill in this fast-paced world. It's a way to protect yourself from stress and overload. Along with "permission" and "enough," "no" is a third word to add to your work–life balance vocabulary.

Rx

- Notice requests that are made of you in the next week—especially when you're squeezed for time.
- Give yourself permission to say No at the next appropriate opportunity.
- Ask for someone else's support and encouragement if you're still not comfortable.
- Decide how you will say No in a diplomatic way.
- Practice ahead of time.

David Posen, M.D.

You can be tactful and still be assertive. You'll be surprised at how free you feel. And it gets easier the more you do it. If you want a role model, just watch any two-year-old the next time he says No to an adult!

Sleep
Don't Leave Home Without It

OW LONG DOES IT TAKE YOU to fall asleep at night? I used to pride myself on being able to fall asleep in a heartbeat. In fact, I used to snap my fingers and say, "I can fall asleep on a dime!" Only recently did I realize that what I was really saying was, "Hey, I'm sleep deprived!" Let me explain ...

As a society, we are shortchanging ourselves on sleep by about sixty to ninety minutes a night. If you wonder whether if you're getting enough, here are seven criteria to help you decide:

- Do you need an alarm clock to wake you up in the morning? Or, two alarm clocks—one close enough to hit the snooze button and one across the room to make you get out of bed?

- Do you wake up feeling refreshed or tired?

- How is your daytime energy? Do you run out of steam by late afternoon?

- How much sleep do you get when you don't have to wake up (on weekends or when you're on vacation)?

- How quickly do you fall asleep at night? This is the criterion used by sleep researchers and it's called the "sleep latency period." For normal, well-rested people, this transition period takes fifteen to twenty minutes. If you fall asleep in less than five minutes—or even ten—you are, by definition, sleep deprived.

When patients complain about fatigue, I always begin by asking two questions:

- How much sleep are you getting at night? The answer is often "six to seven hours."

- How much sleep do you need to function at your best? (Not how much you can get away with, but how much you really need to be at the top of your game.) The answer is usually "eight."

Even a medical student could make the diagnosis: not enough sleep!

How much sleep do we need? Most adults need eight to nine hours a night, which is what people were getting until 1913, when Thomas Edison perfected the tungsten filament incandescent light bulb—artificial

> Many of the symptoms of sleep deprivation are also symptoms of stress.

light. Today we average about seven hours a night, even though we haven't changed physiologically since Edison's time. We're cheating ourselves of sleep in order to work, watch TV, socialize, etc. It hasn't been a very good tradeoff.

WHAT'S THE COST OF SLEEP DEPRIVATION?

The damage is much greater than we realize. We fall asleep while driving; in the United States, 100,000 road accidents a year are attributed to sleepy drivers. We become more prone to infection because our immune system is stimulated during sleep. We make mistakes on the job, causing injury or financial loss. Our concentration and short-term memory are impaired, and intellectual function is diminished. In a *Toronto Star* article on sleep, Dr. Stanley Coren, a psychologist at the University of British Columbia in Vancouver, said, "One hour's lost sleep out of eight results in a drop of one point of IQ and for every additional hour lost, you drop two points. And it accumulates. So if you cheat on sleep by two hours a night over a five-day week, you've lost 15 points." Also, significantly, sleep deprivation affects our mood. We become irritable and depressed.

Note that many of the symptoms of sleep deprivation are also symptoms of stress. But, in addition, tired people are less resilient when handling stressful situations. So lack of sleep is a double whammy. Going to work without proper rest is like starting your day with one foot in a hole.

SLEEP DEBT

The difference between the amount of sleep we need and the amount of sleep we get is called "sleep debt." If you need eight hours a night but only get seven, you have a sleep debt of one hour. As Dr. Coren points out in his wonderful book *Sleep Thieves*, if this continues for a week, you then have an accumulated sleep debt of seven hours. The effect is much like losing all seven hours in the same night. The good news is that you can repay the sleep debt. So if you fall behind, a few consecutive nights of full, uninterrupted sleep will usually return you to full function.

> "I consider the pervasive lack of awareness about sleep deprivation a national emergency."
> William Dement

Five years ago I stopped setting my alarm and simply woke up when my body was ready. Of course, I had to go to bed early enough to wake up naturally and still be on time for work. But the result has been dramatic. I feel profoundly better every day for doing this. And so do my patients who have started getting the sleep they need.

- Assess your sleep situation. How much sleep are you getting now? How much do you need to function at your best? How do you fare with the five sleep criteria?
- Go to bed a half hour earlier for the next few nights and see what happens.
- Then add another half hour for a few nights.
- Continue adding to your sleep until you can wake up naturally, feeling refreshed.
- Sleep in for an hour or two on weekends if you get behind during the week.

David Posen, M.D.

A good night's sleep is the best way to start your day—don't leave home without it!

Caffeine
A Surprisingly Subtle Stressor

TALK ABOUT A STIMULATING birthday party! My wife and I were invited to a restaurant for a fiftieth birthday celebration on a Thursday night. Four couples, lively conversation, wine, some laughs—a fun evening. With appropriate flourish, the birthday cake was served at about 10:30.

This was not your typical cake. It was a chocolate extravaganza that made mud pie look like a tranquilizer. Call it Death by Chocolate. It looked fabulous. My wife and I eyed each other, both with the same thought: is this going to be worth the sleep we'll lose from all that caffeine? We rationalized that we didn't want to offend our hosts, but I wouldn't have passed up that cake for anything! We decided to go for it. And it was as good as it looked.

Then we got home. Midnight came and went. So did 1:00 a.m. We were wired. We finally drifted off about 2:00. And once again I was reminded of the effect of caffeine on stress and sleep.

One intervention, giving up caffeine, has given me the biggest bang for the buck in all my years of stress counseling. Caffeine is such a socially sanctioned substance that we forget it's a drug. It's a stimulant, actually a *strong* stimulant. It stimulates adrenaline release and also blocks a relaxing brain chemical called adenosine. The net result is that it jazzes up your body and produces a stress reaction. I call coffee "stress in a cup."

> Coffee is "stress in a cup."

A study at Duke University showed that people who had two or three cups of coffee in a four-hour period had an adrenaline level 37% higher than the non-coffee-drinking control group. That's a lot of adrenaline chasing around your body for no particular benefit.

I ask all my new patients to try an experiment: to go off caffeine long enough to see if they notice a difference. The period I pick is three weeks. If they feel better without it, they can choose to stay off it; if they *don't* notice a difference they can go back to it.

The results have been dramatic. At least 75% to 80% of my patients feel better without caffeine, and many of them feel dramatically better. I hear testimonials such as: "I can't believe the difference"; "This is incredible"; "Why didn't someone tell me about this earlier?" And most of them stay off it after that, except perhaps for one cup of coffee or tea in the morning.

The benefits include feeling more calm and relaxed, sleeping better and having more energy, less heartburn and less muscle ache. Even participants in my seminars come back to tell me how much better they feel without caffeine.

How about the 20% to 25% who said they didn't notice any difference? When they went back to it, many of them felt a buzz they hadn't noticed before. The effects of caffeine are subtle. The body gets used to it. A colleague who's a microsurgeon told me something interesting. He noticed that, after two cups of coffee, he could see his hand shaking slightly under the microscope, although he couldn't see it with his naked eye. That's how subtle the effects can be.

Caffeine is found in coffee, tea, cola drinks (such as Coke and Pepsi) and chocolate. It is also found in some other soft drinks (Mountain Dew in the United States and Barq's Root Beer, for example) and certain medications, so you have to read labels. Even decaffeinated coffee has a little caffeine in it, so during the experiment I suggest staying off decaf as well.

As if the daytime stress stimulation isn't bad enough, caffeine also messes up your sleep. It can cause insomnia (like that birthday cake). There are lots of people who think it doesn't affect them, but lab studies show that, even if it doesn't keep them awake, caffeine interferes with deep sleep cycles—they get the *quantity* of sleep but not the *quality* they need for optimal rest and rejuvenation.

Caution: Wean yourself off caffeine gradually. If you stop abruptly, you'll get bad, migraine-type withdrawal headaches.

Caffeine gets into your system within minutes, peaks at about an hour and stays in your system six to ten hours (and longer as you get older—one more thing to look forward to). Women on birth control pills take up to eighteen hours to clear caffeine; for pregnant women it's more like twenty-four hours.

And, it accumulates. The coffee you have at supper adds to the caffeine from your mid-afternoon cup of tea and the Coke you have in the evening. That's a lot of caffeine still on board at bedtime.

R_x

- Calculate your daily intake of coffee, tea, cola drinks and chocolate.
- Wean yourself off caffeine gradually. **Don't stop abruptly** or you'll get bad withdrawal migraine headaches. Cut back by one serving each day until you're down to zero.
- If you get a headache, plateau at that level for a few days (or even increase your intake slightly) until the headache goes away. Then start decreasing again.
- Stay off caffeine for three weeks.
- If you start using caffeine again after the experiment, limit yourself to one to two cups a day. And have caffeine only before 12:00 or 1:00 p.m. so it's out of your system by bedtime.

David Posen, M.D.

I avoid caffeine, especially in the evening. But I'm still a pushover for decadent chocolate birthday cakes!

Putting Your Work in Perspective
Step Back and Be Philosophical

W E FINALLY RENTED THE CARTOON feature film *Antz*. If you've ever watched an ant colony and wondered, "What on earth are they doing? What's the point of all this activity?" you're not alone. The main character in the movie, Zee, asked the same question. Voiced by Woody Allen (at his whining, kvetching best), Zee challenged the boring life of a worker ant and aspired to something more. He is an inspiring role model for people who feel like they're on a work treadmill.

Some people literally make work their way of life. Various studies show that one quarter to one third of Canadians consider themselves workaholics. I'm sure they're not all thrilled with this life of constant toil, but they've allowed work to fill their time, pervade their thoughts and obscure the other parts of their existence. A recent book title sums it up: *The Man Who Mistook his Job for a Life*. When you're a hammer, everything looks like a nail; when you're a drone, everything looks like work. Ask Zee the ant.

> We are finite individuals trying to do open-ended jobs. But we're limited by our physiology.

There are two ways to reduce the feeling of stress from an all-consuming job. One is to reorganize your work—reduce the hours and get more balance in your life. The other is to *think* about your work differently. Instead of getting resentful, put it in perspective. Here are some thoughts to consider:

- **You're here by choice.** Unless a press gang dragged you from a local tavern in a drunken stupor (the way they "recruited" British sailors in the seventeenth century), you chose your job. And you *reaffirm* that choice every day you show up for work.

- **You're not alone.** Look around. Most people are feeling overloaded and occasionally overwhelmed. There's nothing wrong with you! Everyone in today's workplace is struggling.

- **You can only do so much.** We are finite individuals trying to do open-ended jobs. But we're limited by our physiology. There's only so much you can do. Modify your expectations—you can't do it all. Stop trying.

- **Focus on the positives of your job.** People work for more than a paycheck. What else do you get from your job? Benefits include stimulation, challenge, new learning, relationships, camaraderie, variety, excitement and finding meaning and significance in how your work affects others. When you get dispirited, step back and remind yourself of all the things you *like* about your job.

- **Focus on what's there, not on what's missing.** When there's an endless amount of work, it's easy to feel unfulfilled and frustrated because you haven't finished everything. In the new workplace it's virtually impossible to ever finish—and even if you do, there are other value-added tasks you can pursue. Instead of feeling discouraged and berating yourself for the things that you didn't do or finish, acknowledge yourself at the end of each day for what you've accomplished. Phrases like "That was a really productive day" and "I got a lot done today" will help to shift the emphasis.

- **You are more than your job.** As people spend more time at work, they start to identify with their job, role or title. Workers define themselves as "I'm a teacher, I'm a manager, I'm an IT specialist." Even worse, many folks *over*-identify with their jobs to an extent where they *become* their job title. Remind yourself that you are not your job and your job is not your life. Your work is only what you *do*, not who you *are*.

> "Words and thoughts are the weapons against stress."
> J. Clayton Lafferty

- **Step away from your work and discover there's a life beyond it.** The best way to get perspective on your job is to step back from it. I can always see my work clearer from a distance—especially when I'm on vacation. Not that I dwell on work while I'm away (and if I did, I wouldn't write about it in a book about balancing your life!). But little insights and helpful ideas pop into my head on occasion when I'm in a totally different environment.

You can get perspective by going for a walk in the country or taking an evening off to go to the symphony. Reflect on the life you've created and put it in context, or fix it—or both. (You may even admit that you're in the wrong job and it's time for a change.)

Rx

- Set aside one to two hours this week to get completely away from work. Go down to the waterfront, sit by a fire or go for a long walk or a drive in the country.
- Ask yourself what you like most about your job—and about your non-work life.
- What things aren't working out so well? (What would you like to change?)
- Pick one item to work on, one change, big or small, that you can make this week to improve your situation.
- At the end of each day, reflect on and acknowledge what you enjoyed and what you accomplished.

David Posen, M.D.

Zee had the pluck to envision a better life, and the courage to seek it out. If a little ant can do that, there's hope for everyone. Let him be a beacon for us all.

How to Leave Work at Work

They Don't Pay You for Twenty-Four Hours a Day

YOU KNOW YOU'RE IN LOVE when you can't stop thinking about your beloved. So what does it mean when you can't stop thinking about work? That you love your job? Probably not. That your employers are paying you megabucks to buy not only your daytime effort but also "air time" in your head at night? If only you were paid so well! (And how much would they have to pay to buy your thoughts around the clock?) Yet something's causing your mind to revert to work like the default setting on a computer.

Many people tell me that work thoughts often intrude upon their off-hours. The ultimate example is when they wake up in the middle of the night with their minds already in gear—especially if they have trouble *turning off* the thoughts.

There was a time when people went to work, put in their hours, clocked out and forgot about work until the next day. They maintained a healthy separation between work and family/personal time. Today's work hours are less well defined. The line has blurred at the work–life interface and we're taking work home literally (in our briefcases) and figuratively (in our heads). It's taking over our lives.

> The time has come to establish boundaries, to keep work in its place and to make room for important relationships and activities.

The time has come to establish boundaries, to keep work in its place and to make room for important relationships and activities—even for down time to just relax. Here are some suggestions for leaving work at the office:

- **Don't bring work home.** You can't do it if you don't lug it home to begin with. When you bring it home, two things can happen: either it sucks you into work-related activity or it sits there, rebuking you: "Hey, what about *me*?"

- **Get unplugged at home.** The good news about technology is that people can reach you anywhere. The bad news about technology is that people can reach you anywhere. Turn off all your tech gadgets and clear the decks so that evenings and weekends are for other things (like Nintendo, computer games and DVD movies. Okay, amend that to say turn off the *work-related* technology!)

- **Have a life to go to after work.** I arranged to have something delivered to me, and the person offered to bring it over on the weekend. I said I didn't want to intrude on her personal time, to which she replied, "Oh, that's okay, I have no life, anyway." She said it with a smile, but it really saddened me. Develop compelling activities and enjoyable relationships that will entice you in your free time. In other words, "Get a life."

> We're better at compartmentalizing our thinking than we give ourselves credit for.

- **Shut off your thinking about work.** Compartmentalize. Discipline yourself to keep your mind from wandering onto work subjects when you're away from the office. Find diversion and distraction.

- **Park your problems.** A patient told me she visualizes putting her work problems on a shelf when she gets home and not taking them off the shelf until she's ready to leave for work the next day. How's that for discipline? But she could have gone one step further, and put them on a shelf when she left work, not picking them up until she arrived at the office the next day.

- **Organize your next day's schedule before you leave.** It's a good time to plan because everything is fresh, and you know what priorities you're working on. Then you can tune out and free up your mind for other things. You'll have a sense of completion at the end of the day and be able to hit the ground running the next day.

- **Create decompression or buffer time between work and home.** This is what the Brits do when they drop into their local pub on the way home to grab a pint and a few laughs. Stop off at the gym or meet a friend. Or, when you get home, go for a walk or have a hot bath before starting to prepare dinner.

- **Change your clothes when you get home.** As one of my patients put it, "As long as I'm wearing this suit, I feel like I'm still at work." Changing into more comfortable clothes creates separation and helps to create a relaxed mindset for the evening.

- Start leaving your briefcase, laptop and professional reading at the office.
- Stop making work-related phone calls and handling voice mail or e-mail on your own time.
- If a problem (or even a solution or good idea) pops into your head at home, write it down quickly and put it away. Don't act on it until you return to the office.
- Write out your next day's schedule before leaving work.
- Clean off (or organize) your desk at the end of each day, even if you haven't finished all your tasks.

David Posen, M.D.

For most of us, the work week is long enough. Let's not extend the hours. And who knows? If you work less, you just might end up loving your job more.

Reclaiming Ownership
of Your Time
A Little Goes a Long Way

W HEN I INTERNED IN EDMONTON, Alberta, I found an hour a day I'd never had before. As a student at the University of Toronto for six years, I'd lived about half an hour from campus. This meant commuting for an hour or more every day. I never gave it much thought. It was just part of my life.

But when I got to Edmonton, I lived in the house staff residence 50 yards from the hospital. I quickly discovered something amazing: I could leave for work at 7:58 and arrive a minute early. When I left at 6:00 p.m. I was home at 6:01. Living beside the hospital gave me an extra hour every day. It was an hour I've never given up since! After that year, I determined to live no more than ten minutes from my work—and I've kept that promise. In terms of work–life balance, it's been a tremendous benefit.

Over my last fourteen years of general practice, my office hours fluctuated. I began with a workday of 8:00 a.m. to 6:00 p.m., which gradually expanded to 7:00 p.m. When our first child was born, I decided to leave the office at 6:00 again and thus gave myself an hour a day I had not had in years.

I was cheating myself by an hour a day.

Work–life balance has become difficult for most of us. It involves several juggling acts, the first of which is balancing the time devoted to work with the time away from work. I diagram this as a pie in which the work–life proportions are roughly 60/40. If you can move the line slightly to the left, it will give you more time on the "life" or "non-work" side of the pie (see chart on page 75).

Surprisingly, a little goes a long way. Dr. Juliet Schor did the math in her wonderful book *The Overworked American*. I've summarized her findings in the following diagram:

Work—Life Balance
"The 1st Juggling Act"

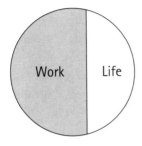 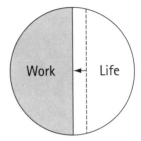

48 minutes/day

= 4 hours/week

= 200 hours/year (based on a 50-week year)

= 4 weeks/year (based on a 50-hour week)

= 1 month/year

This means that, by cutting your work hours by just under an hour a day, over a year you gain a month's worth of discretionary time for other uses. (This does not mean that if you stay those extra forty-eight minutes each day you can take off the month of August—but I'm still working on that one!) An aggregate of a month's worth of time per year, every year, is not something to sneeze at.

Leaving work a little earlier requires some organization and planning. But it's mostly a matter of discipline and determination. And the payoff is huge.

Many of my patients have enjoyed the experience of reclaiming ownership of their time. One was an executive who was putting in ten-hour days on top of her hour-long commute twice a day. So her work day was twelve hours, door to door. She came to see me because she was stressed and exhausted (no surprise there). She said, "I know I'm not productive with such long hours, but it's a Catch 22." I suggested that she leave the office an hour earlier as an experiment.

Three weeks later she reported, "It's better by far. And I still accomplish the same amount of work." She summed it up by saying "I was cheating myself by an hour a day."

Another patient had a workaholic boss who seemed to have no life away from the office. After putting in long evenings and many weekends for months, the patient finally drew the line and stopped making himself available after-hours. He took back a piece of his life that he'd given away to please a boss who cared more about face time and meetings than the well-being of his employees.

> If you don't take control of your time, someone else will.

Obviously, many people have to work evenings and/or weekend shifts. But many others have allowed their work to creep unnecessarily into these sanctums of family and personal time. It is this group that can "take back their lives" if they choose.

Rx
- Estimate the number of hours per week you're working now. Write down the number.
- Then track your hours over the next few days (including commuting time and work done from home) and calculate your hours per week.

Are you working more hours than you thought?

- Next week, make an arbitrary decision to leave work thirty to forty-five minutes earlier (or start later). Stick to your guns.
- Re-evaluate after three weeks and cut back again if you're still working more than nine hours a day.
- Start protecting evenings and weekends as "work-free zones" in your schedule. This includes ignoring or closing e-mail and just watching for personal messages—for example on Facebook.

David Posen, M.D.

While living at the house staff residence in Edmonton, I learned a lot about the importance of reclaiming my time. But that residence was good to me in another way: I also learned to shoot pool in my recreational time—a skill that still serves me well on occasion.

Making Time for Leisure

How to Make Time When There Isn't Any Time

"I'M OVERWHELMED. I DON'T SLEEP. I can't take this." That is how Barbara felt about the many responsibilities in her life. She was a manager in a large organization and had a young child at home. She wanted help to "get more things done and to be more organized." At the end of our first visit, I recommended that she read my book *Always Change a Losing Game*, and we agreed to meet three weeks later.

Upon her return, she reported that she'd come to a profound realization: "I've been asking the wrong question," she said. "Instead of asking 'How can I do more?' I should be asking 'Why am I trying to do so much?'" She had been devoting 90% of her time and energy to her paid job and home chores, and minimal time to herself. She decided to cut back on her work hours (she was putting in a lot of unpaid overtime) to spend more time with her daughter and pursue one of her great loves, reading. When she changed her schedule, her stress level diminished and her enjoyment of each day increased.

Leisure is in short supply in our busy lives. Increasing numbers of people are spending their free time doing chores, running errands and grocery shopping.

What can we do about this situation? How can we make time for leisure when there doesn't seem to be enough time? First, as Barbara did, we need to change our philosophy and our priorities. One way to make the time is to *give yourself permission* to do things for yourself and *make them a priority*.

> "Identify your values and support them behaviorally."
> Dr. Roger Mellott

Dr. Roger Mellott, a stress consultant in Louisiana, was once asked to summarize the essence of stress management in one sentence. He did it in seven words: "Identify your values and support them behaviorally." Decide what's important to you, and then live in a way that's consistent with those values.

Here are some other suggestions that will help you make time for leisure:

- **Rotate your values.** Work is a primary value for most of us. In fact, we give it most of our best time and energy. Family is also a primary value. Dr. Mellott suggests "rotating your values" as a way to make time for things that are important. When he returns from business trips, where work is the focus, he shifts gears and makes family his primary focus.

  > Do something for yourself every day.

  But we also need to make time for *ourselves*. My motto is "Do something for yourself every day" (for at least an hour on weekdays and two hours on weekend days). It doesn't have to be all at once. You might go for a half-hour walk at lunchtime and read for thirty minutes in the evening.

- **Combine your values.** I knew a couple of avid golfers who had children aged six and eight. They devised a creative way of combining those two loves: they took their children golfing with them. But the kids weren't just spectators. Each went with a parent on a golf cart. The parents drove off the tees and played the fairways; the kids putted the greens. The result was a family outing in which the parents pursued their passion for golf, while spending fun time with their kids.

- **Trade money for time.** Another way to make time for leisure is to buy it. Hiring someone to cut the grass, shovel the snow, clean your house or babysit your kids will buy you valuable time to unwind, play tennis or meet a friend. I take the train into Toronto instead of driving because it affords me time to read or relax. Buy a second refrigerator to store food bought in bulk—then shop less often. Takeout food or delivery can save you cooking time, which can be used for other pursuits.

  > "I have a microwave fireplace. You can lay down in front of the fire all night in eight minutes."
  > Steven Wright

- **Learn to take shortcuts.** Beds don't have to be made with hospital corners. You don't have to iron sheets or T-shirts. Snow shoveling only has to be expedient; it doesn't have to be a work of art.

- **Overcome guilt.** Leisure is not a luxury, it's a necessity. It's crucial for health, energy, productivity and reducing stress. Think of how you use your leisure moments: exercising, playing sports, spending time with family and friends, relaxing, reading, listening to (or playing) music, doing hobbies. What laws or moral codes are broken by these activities? There's nothing to feel guilty about.

Rx

- Pick one leisure activity you'd like to make time for. Decide how often you can realistically do it in an average week.
- Choose the best time to do it (a crossword puzzle over lunch, a run after work).
- Make a date with yourself to start this week.
- Write it into your schedule or BlackBerry.
- Refute guilt messages. Remind yourself that you need the leisure time to maintain your physical and mental health. Better yet, remind yourself how hard you work—you deserve a break.

David Posen, M.D.

Barbara found balance and leisure by listening to her instincts and living in a way consistent with her values. It's a formula worth following.

Beliefs That Oppose Balance and Leisure
The Hidden Rules That Run Your Life

"HOW MANY OF YOU FEEL comfortable getting up from dinner on a summer evening and going for a walk or a bike ride before you clean up the kitchen and wash the dishes?" This is the question I posed at one of my work–life balance seminars. A few liberated souls put up their hands, but most people felt uncomfortable with the idea. (A few even shuddered at the notion.) We then explored the thinking behind this reluctance. We discovered it was based on a series of beliefs they held about work and leisure—the most basic of which was "work should come before pleasure." As we probed deeper, someone blurted out, "My house has to be clean before I can enjoy myself." As soon as she said it, she registered a look of surprise at her own discovery. This message had been in her mind (and guiding her behavior) for years without her ever being aware of it until that moment.

> We hold our beliefs to be "the Truth"—so they become the Truth for us.

Notice the certainty with which the remark was made—like it was some fundamental, unassailable fact of life. This is what makes belief systems so fascinating.

Here's why beliefs are so powerful:

1. Beliefs are premises and assumptions that we hold about how things should be, how people should behave and how the world works.

2. We generally hold our beliefs subconsciously, unaware of them and their power over us. In fact, they're *more* powerful because they're hidden from view.

3. We hold our beliefs to be "the Truth"—therefore they *become* the Truth for us.

4. Beliefs guide and often dictate our behavior and decisions. They literally run our lives. (And you thought it was your mother, your boss and your homeroom teacher!)

Over the years, I've collected a list of beliefs that oppose balance and leisure. Most of the people who made these claims were surprised to hear themselves stating rules and regulations about how to live that seemed to come out of nowhere:

GENERAL BELIEFS

- You have to meet other people's needs before you meet your own.

- If you want something done right, you have to do it yourself.

- You have to finish everything every day.

- You should always be busy.

- Leisure is a luxury.

- You have to be all things to all people.

- Sleep is for wimps.

- A woman's work is never done.

- If it's worth doing, it's worth doing right.

- You shouldn't watch TV during the day (even on weekends).

WORK-RELATED BELIEFS

- If you don't work hard and work long hours, you won't get ahead.

- Hard work + money = success.

- Being seen = commitment.

- I don't need breaks.

- Saying No is not acceptable and, therefore, not an option.

- To ask for help is a weakness.

- If your boss is there, you should be there.

- I need to be available 24/7.

- Being a "work martyr" is a badge of honor.

- Do whatever it takes (to deliver, to get ahead, to succeed).

These are real statements from real people. It's no wonder that balance and leisure are in short supply.

Phrases that include "should," "need to," "have to" or "must" are usually beliefs. Generalizations and judgments, such as "People who leave early are slackers," are also beliefs. The problem with beliefs is they often don't serve us very well. To take more control of our lives and create better balance, we need to do three things (oops, that's stated as yet another "belief." How about "I suggest we do three things?"):

"Everybody should believe in something—
—I believe I'll have another drink"
Unknown

1. Identify our beliefs that oppose balance and leisure.

2. Challenge those beliefs. Stop accepting them as the truth. Hold them up to the light and look at them critically. Beliefs are not the truth but simply *our version* of the truth, our opinions about things.

3. Revise the beliefs that are limiting us and replace them with new ones (or expand them to be more inclusive and less rigid). Here are some examples of more constructive beliefs:

- It's okay, even desirable, to make time for yourself each day.

- Leisure is not a luxury, it's a necessity for good health, energy and workplace productivity.

- There are times when it's okay—even necessary—to say No.

- Taking breaks actually improves work performance.

- It's possible to meet my own needs as well as the needs of others. I can do both.

- Other people can do things as well as I can—sometimes even better (or, at least, well enough).

- This week, start to notice your priorities—the order in which you do things—and observe how your belief systems may be influencing your daily choices.

- Start to ask questions that will reveal your hidden beliefs ("Why am I working long hours?", "Why am I doing house chores when I'd rather be outside?", etc.)

- Try to determine where these beliefs came from or who taught them to you.

- Talk to people whose balance you admire. Find out what beliefs are supporting them.

- Pick one belief to revise or reword so that it supports balance in your life (for example, change "work before pleasure" to "work in addition to pleasure").

David Posen, M.D.

The woman in my seminar who stated "My house has to be clean before I can enjoy myself" walked away that day with a smile of profound discovery, determined to question and replace the "rules" that were running her life.

Pacing and Time-Outs
Even PVRs Have a Pause Button

DURING MY INTERNSHIP IN 1967, I was assisting at a late-morning gall bladder operation. Near the end, when the surgeon and resident didn't need me anymore, I said I was going to have lunch. They started to laugh and needle me. Unknowingly, I'd broken the protocol that everyone stayed until the operation was over. However, I was hungry and tired, we were starting outpatient clinic at 1:00, and I felt in need of a break. But that story followed me for the rest of the year, getting wilder with every telling.

Taking breaks increases our efficiency and productivity—and reduces stress. Time-outs are built into every sport, from half-time in football to side changes in tennis. Physical laborers take time-outs, and everyone understands their need to rest muscles and regain energy. But most of us today are knowledge workers, and too many people think nothing of working from 8:00 to 6:00 without even stopping for lunch. Bad idea! Mental work is also tiring. We fool ourselves if we think we can do it well without taking time-outs. In my work–life balance seminars, I often ask how many participants can listen to a two-hour lecture without once losing focus, or read work-related material for two hours and retain total attention? I've yet to see a hand go up.

> Periodic breaks actually increase your productivity and pay you back for the time taken.

The need for periodic breaks is supported by science. Dr. Ernest Rossi, in his excellent book *The 20-Minute Break*, explains that we have two-hour cycles throughout the day in which our energy and activity levels rise, peak and then come down. Then our bodies go into a state of physiological rest for about twenty minutes.

Dr. Rossi calls these "ultradian" cycles and advocates taking "ultradian healing breaks." He suggests that, because our productivity is reduced anyway, we should use these twenty-minute periods for rest and recovery. My own productivity has been enhanced considerably by this kind of pacing.

How do you know when you need a break? Our bodies give us signals. The most obvious sign is fatigue. Or our brains just shut down—we lose our concentration. Or we feel restless and need to stretch or move around. Unfortunately, most people ignore these signals and keep soldiering on. It's better to pay attention and take a short intermission. If you can't take twenty minutes, take ten (or even five).

Now, you can't always take a break when the feeling hits you. After all, if you're sitting in a meeting it's hard to say, "Oops, I just got a signal from my body that it's time for a breather. See you later." We just have to time it the best we can.

> Conferences and seminars always have breaks built into the schedule. If they didn't, who would show up on the second day?

You may be wondering, "How can I take a twenty-minute break every two hours when I'm already overloaded with work?" The ironic thing is that periodic breaks actually increase your productivity and pay you back for the time taken. They're a smart investment. And it's not that big a deal to take them. The traditional schedule of morning and afternoon "coffee" breaks plus time for lunch pretty much divides your day into ultradian cycles.

The benefits of time-outs are not restricted to restoring energy. Breaks are also important for reducing stress and for stepping back to reflect on your work—they provide contemplation time to get perspective on tough problems. When I do counseling, I need a break between sessions to clear my head and get ready for the next patient.

There are lots of ways to take a break. A friend of mine calls these "snapshot vacations." Any of the following will help:

- a power nap (five to twenty minutes)

- meditation or relaxation exercises (see pages 162–64)

- daydreaming

- a nutrition break (eat lunch or a high-energy, low-fat snack)

- a walk or other physical activity

- a music break (radio or iPod)

- a social break (phone a friend or visit a colleague down the hall—of course, your "intermission" might be their "interruption")
- a bathroom break (perhaps the only place where people will leave you alone for a few minutes)
- a humor break (a book of cartoons or a comedy tape)
- a hobby break (a crossword puzzle or solitaire)
- a reading break (a magazine article or book)
- a sunshine break—go outside for some rays and fresh air
- low-concentration tasks—sometimes a change is as good as a rest: sort through your mail, do some photocopying, return a phone call

Rx

- Look at your present schedule. Do you take breaks during the day?
- Plan to take at least one break a day—at least for lunch. Decide the best time for you. Write it into your schedule.
- Choose the kind of break that would work best for you.
- Start to monitor your body and your performance. Notice when your energy and mental concentration start to flag. Keep track on paper for a few days to see if there's a pattern.
- Give yourself permission to take short "ad hoc" breaks when you feel yourself winding down. A two-minute walk down the hall may be all you need to perk up.

David Posen, M.D.

Taking time-outs is an important way to pace yourself. Humans are not built to work non-stop. Even PVRs have a pause button! So take a tip from technology, and give yourself a break.

It's Time to Plan
Your Next Vacation

"I Could Never Accomplish in Twelve Months
What I Can Get Done in Eleven!"

A CEO BOUNCED INTO MY OFFICE recently—sun-tanned, and with a big smile and an air of calm about him. He'd just returned from a relaxing family vacation during which he called his office only once. He didn't take an alarm clock and by the fourth day he was sleeping eight hours a night. He now plans to take five weeks of vacation a year (instead of his previous two or three). Another convert to the importance of vacations.

Spring is a great time of year to be a stress counselor. Most of my patients feel better at that time of year. I wish I could take credit for this sudden collective improvement, but I know there are two other factors making a difference: the days are getting longer and the weather warmer; and many people are just back from March vacations, and feel refreshed and invigorated.

As a self-employed person, I've always been amazed at salaried people who don't take their full allotment of paid vacation time. If you're such a person, I have three words of advice: Stop Doing That! If someone paid me to stay away, I wouldn't keep showing up at the office to work for free. Take all you're entitled to. Even if you just stay home and sit under a tree.

> Take your holidays before you need them. Then you'll never need them. You'll just enjoy them.

Just as we need time-outs during the day to restore our energy and concentration, we need longer amounts of time off throughout the year to really get away, clear our heads, pursue other interests, and reconnect with family and friends.

Why don't people take regular vacations? I've heard all the excuses over the years: "I can't get away from work"; "I'm just too busy"; "No one else can do my job"; "It's too much of a hassle to go away—extra work before I leave and a pile of work when I get back"; "I don't have enough money"; "I don't have anybody to go away with"; "If I leave, they may realize they can get along without me." More subtly, people may feel more important if they're too busy to go away. They may believe that holidays are for wimps. Or they may harbor a subconscious belief that vacations are luxuries, or a waste of time.

I have a motto: Take your holidays before you need them. Then you'll never need them, you'll just enjoy them. Don't wait until you're so depleted that your vacation turns into a convalescence. Be proactive. Take timely vacations while you still have some energy to enjoy yourself. I learned this lesson in the 1970s when I went eight months without a vacation. Finally, I planned a trip. But three weeks before my departure, I hit the wall. I needed a break—immediately! I booked off the next week and just hung around home relaxing. Two weeks later I took my planned excursion. When you have to take time off to prepare for your time off, you've waited too long. I never did that again.

> "Where do forest rangers go to 'get away from it all?'"
> George Carlin

Vacations don't have to be expensive to be beneficial. My best vacations are spent out of town, but even taking time off to stay home can be relaxing and enjoyable if you curtail your regular routine. Sleep in, read a novel, walk along the lake or take a drive in the country. Go on day trips or visit friends. There are also ways to travel inexpensively: visit friends, travel on frequent-flyer points or go camping at government-run campgrounds.

Vacations are good for the body and good for the soul. If you do a vacation right, you come back feeling refreshed and eager to return to work. As one man put it, "I could never accomplish in twelve months what I can get done in eleven!"

Here are some tips:

- Plan to take all the vacation time your employer allows. If you're self-employed, give yourself at least two to three breaks a year.

- Spread your vacation time over the year (instead of taking it all at once.) As soon as you return from a holiday, plan the next one.

- Organize your work so other people can cover for you while you're away.

- Don't take work-related material with you. This includes professional reading, laptops and smartphones. If you feel naked without that stuff, it's a chance to break your dependency—an added benefit!

- Don't call the office, and don't tell them where they can reach you. Make it a clean break.

- Come home a day early to ease the transition into full work mode.

- Plan a light first day back to work (for catch-up and readjustment).

Rx

- Look at your calendar. Book off time for your next vacation.
- Decide where you want to go and with whom. Coordinate your schedules.
- Or plan to stay home—but arrange enjoyable, pleasurable activities. (Don't use the time to do home renovations or to catch up on work).
- Pick up your phone and make some reservations this week.

David Posen, M.D.

I applauded my CEO patient for his new vacation philosophy and made one suggestion: "Next time, don't call your office even once!"

Burnout

The Best Treatment Is Prevention

JOE WAS A TALENTED, bright executive in a large company. He was also a prime candidate for burnout: a workaholic, Type-A perfectionist who expected himself to know everything and take care of everyone. And he was a pleaser who hated confrontation. This combination of conscientiousness, obsessiveness and reluctance to let anybody down created a lot of stress in his life.

At work he was meticulous, worked long hours and took everything seriously. Office politics, a difficult boss and a lot of travel certainly didn't help. He had few outside interests other than his family.

As things got more difficult, Joe pedaled harder and faster. He worked even longer hours and went in on weekends, cutting back on family time and exercise. Then he developed insomnia and other stress symptoms. Through it all he maintained his unrealistically high standards of performance, not wanting to let anyone down nor look bad to his staff. He thought he could do everything if he just worked harder. But the more he struggled, the more difficult things got. And the more difficult they got, the harder he pushed himself. Finally, he wore himself out, had to be hospitalized briefly, required anti-depressant medication and had to take an extended leave of absence from work.

Burnout is a big problem, and it's dramatic when it happens. Grown men can be reduced to tears. Dr. Herbert Freudenberger's classic book *Burn-out* defines burnout this way: "To deplete oneself. To exhaust one's physical and mental resources. To wear oneself out by excessively striving to reach some *unrealistic* expectation imposed by one's self or by the values of society" (I've added the italics for emphasis). He calls burnout the "super-achiever sickness." Freudenberger states, "Whenever the expectation level is dramatically opposed to reality and the person persists in trying to reach that expectation, trouble is on the way."

> The burnout sequence begins with high ideals and expectations.

The burnout sequence begins with high ideals and expectations: a teacher who's going to inspire every student, a nurse who's going to save every life, a lawyer who's going to win every case or a therapist who's going to cure every client. People in the helping professions are particularly prone to burnout. So are business executives with high levels of ambition who are prepared to do whatever it takes to become "successful" (in whatever way they actually measure that).

The sequence continues when these people put out a high amount of energy to pursue their goals. If their efforts produce rewards (praise, promotions, raises, satisfaction), all well and good. But if they don't get the expected rewards, instead of stepping back to reevaluate their goals, potential burnout candidates simply increase their efforts. If the expected reward is still not forthcoming, symptoms start to appear.

Dr. Freudenberger describes three stages of burnout, which I've summarized in this chart:

Stage I (early): *Fatigue,* decreased performance, stress symptoms

Stage I (later): *Exhaustion,* frustration, disillusionment

Stage II: *Denial,* impaired judgment, blaming others, defensiveness, apathy, cynicism, depression

Stage III: Disorientation, despondency, despair, disengagement, distancing, "dullness and deadness."

This is a terrible spiral to be in. The whole process usually takes years, but there are many warning signs that are missed along the way. The main factors contributing to burnout are:

- unrealistic expectations (especially perfectionism and idealism)

- over identifying with job, career, title or cause

- single-minded pursuit of goals

- limited interests and activities beyond the area of focus

It's best not to get caught in the burnout spiral in the first place. You can prevent it through balance, energy management and realistic expectations:

- **Balance prevents burnout.** I've never seen burnout in anybody who had other activities and meaningful relationships in their lives. Involvement with family and friends, and activities such as exercise and hobbies all prevent burnout.

- **Monitor and manage your energy.** This is extremely important. Fatigue and exhaustion are Stage I symptoms of burnout. Get enough sleep, eat well and exercise regularly. Be aware if your energy level is low or getting worse.

- **Realistic expectations are critical.** Whatever your field, recognize that everything won't always go smoothly. You won't move steadily up the success ladder. Teachers won't reach every student; patients will die in spite of the best efforts of the most dedicated doctors and nurses. Not every talented athlete will become a professional or champion. We need to regularly evaluate our goals and expectations and do a reality check so that we don't over-invest our time and effort in quests that will be futile. It's disappointing enough when things don't work out as you planned. But if you cling to unrealistic goals, failure to reach them will be devastating.

If you, or someone you know, are showing symptoms of early burnout or depression, seek professional help as quickly as possible.

Rx ● This week, step back and think about your career goals and expectations. Are they realistic? How are you handling setbacks and disappointments? (Philosophically? Fearfully? With a desperate need to redouble your efforts? With determination to succeed at all costs?)

- Monitor your energy level each day (rate it on a scale of 1 to 5 or "high, medium, low"). Keep a chart for a few days. Look for other symptoms of stress and/or depression.
- Look at your schedule. Are you making time for exercise, relationships, hobbies and other non-work activities? If not, add one of these to your calendar this week—and cut back on one work activity.
- If you're exhausted, reduce your work hours and schedule time for more sleep, relaxation and leisure activity.

David Posen, M.D.

Joe got over his Stage II burnout and depression. He returned to work, but never stayed past 6:00. He also took a vacation. In our last conversation, he said, "I've cut way back on my work hours—and it's amazing. I'm doing more at work in less time—and it seems a lot more fun too." This burnout story finally had a happy ending, but it would have been better if it hadn't happened at all. Don't let it happen to you.

> Sometimes we have to deal with disappointment philosophically, instead of refusing to accept reality.

Dealing with Deadlines
Finding Flexibility—and Gender Language

A N AUTHOR TOLD ME AN INTERESTING story. His book was nearing completion and he was casting around for endorsement quotes for the cover. He was given a deadline to obtain these quotes, but was having trouble getting dynamite material. The deadline got closer. His publisher kept calling. Then he got one excellent testimonial, which took some of the heat off. But they needed a second one. He was running out of time as well as luck.

Finally, a best-selling author agreed to review his manuscript. His hopes rose, his publisher started salivating and suddenly the deadline wasn't so rigid—in fact it was extended by more than a week. Magically, the publisher was able to find an extra ten days in the printing schedule.

Most of us find deadlines a source of pressure or even intimidation. But most deadlines are arbitrary. It's fascinating that they hold such power over us. One reason might be contained in the word "deadline" itself. I looked it up in *Webster's Dictionary* and found it was originally a military term: "A line drawn around a prison, to cross which involves for a prisoner the liability of being instantly shot. Hence, a fixed limit, beyond which disaster is imminent." If that doesn't scare you, you're made of tougher stuff than I am!

We seem to think of deadlines as holding potentially fatal consequences for us if they aren't met.

Someone later told me more about the background. Apparently, the word was coined during the American Civil War. Soldiers were on the move, so if they took prisoners they had no jails to put them in. The custom was to assemble prisoners in one place and draw a line on the ground to mark the perimeter of the detainment area. The captives were told that if they stayed within the designated area they would be protected—but if they crossed over the "dead" line, they would be fired on. This was serious stuff!

The word was later borrowed by the publishing industry, as noted in Webster's: "The hour at which the printing forms of a newspaper are locked, after which no copy can be inserted. Hence, the time set as a limit for completion of any operation. The latest time by which something must be done." Doesn't that sound benevolent compared to the military usage? We seem to think of deadlines as holding potentially fatal consequences for us if they aren't met. I think it's time to rethink the concept.

Deadlines are almost always more flexible than we think. I've seen theater performances start late because important people are not yet in their seats. I was recently on a plane where the departure was delayed because of late-boarding passengers.

Here are some thoughts about managing deadlines:

- Don't accept or promise what you can't deliver. Communicate your concerns and negotiate a time that's realistic.

- If you're unsure whether you can meet a target date, accept the work conditionally and express your reservations. It's better to under-promise and over-deliver than the other way around.

- Calculate a realistic time frame—and then add a cushion! Don't make your schedule too tight. Leave room for interruptions and unforeseen events such as computer glitches.

- Plan ahead. Organize. Schedule the work. Break the task into component parts, with time frames for each.

- Start early. Don't procrastinate.

- Avoid perfectionism, especially early in the project. You can always fine-tune later if there's time.

- If you're behind schedule, brainstorm options with your boss. You might ask your boss to

  — get you extra help

  — relieve you of other duties

- scale back the scope of the project

- reprioritize the task, and decide which elements are essential and which can wait.

- help you determine the preferred delivery date and the point of no return (the real deadline).

- Keep people up to date with regular progress reports. If you're running behind schedule, inform them as soon as possible. Don't wait till the eleventh hour to deliver bad news.

Obviously, we need time limits and target dates to keep things moving. There's nothing like a little time urgency to get procrastinators going. But let's stop living as if these deadlines were literal swords hanging over our heads.

R𝗑
- Start using more moderate language ("time frame," "time limit," or "target date") instead of the scary "deadline."
- Look at your current schedule. List the projects and tasks that have a definite completion date. Note the target date beside each item. Arrange them chronologically.
- Start working on the one with the nearest due date.
- Set out a schedule for completion of the work. Aim to finish before the absolute zero hour.
- Peruse the other projects and list the resources and supplies you'll need. Arrange to get them ahead of time.

David Posen, M.D.

My author friend got a glowing endorsement from the best-selling author, which helped to launch his new book. Since the original deadline hadn't been as fixed as first stated, everyone was pleased!

Prioritizing Tasks
The Art of Doing First Things First

HANG AROUND ANY BUSY EMERGENCY room and you will see something very instructive. Since ERs are always open, they can be inundated without warning. Unpredictability is the norm, and the potential for chaos is high. There needs to be a system to make sure the sickest patients are seen first. That's why emergency rooms have "triage nurses," who prioritize incoming patients based on how urgent their need for treatment is.

When I worked in emergency rooms, we'd have an assortment of ailments to deal with: heart attack, abdominal pain, asthma, fractures, lacerations, earaches. The variety was fascinating. The nurses and I were constantly adjusting our priorities to attend to people with life-threatening problems first, patients in severe pain second, people who might require surgery third, and so on. We also had the occasional intoxicated person making a big fuss to be seen for some minor scrape. It was an exercise in prioritizing in which the stakes were high, as were the emotions.

Triage is a classic illustration of "first things first," but the same principle applies in all workplaces. Overload is a constant for working people. With all the demands on our plates each day, organization becomes a never-ending challenge. Thus the urgent need to prioritize!

> If you deal with tasks before they are urgent, they'll never actually become urgent.

Watch successful people, and you'll notice they don't spend much time on trivial items. They work on the things that are most important. But how do they decide what's important? For some, decisions are driven by deadlines; for others, they're based on what's important to their boss, what will earn them the most money, or what will bring them closer to their personal goals.

Whatever your criteria, consider what matters most and make decisions accordingly. It helps to have a system. The following two models have stood the test of time. The first is Alan Lakein's model from his classic book *How to Get Control of Your Time and Your Life.* It's sometimes called the "ABC System." First, make a To Do list of tasks you want or need to accomplish. Then label each item: "A" for things that must be done, "B" for things that should be done, and "C" for things that may be done, if there's time. (The Cs are discretionary. Most of the time, you probably won't get to them.)

Once you've identified the importance of each task, do the A priority tasks first. (Remember: "first things first.") The problem for many of us is that we like to do the Cs first: they're often quick, easy—even fun—and they provide a feeling of satisfaction. However, they're often just a way of putting off the important things (which may be onerous and less pleasant). But if you discipline yourself to do the highest priority tasks first, the rest of the day goes much more easily and enjoyably.

Once you've done the As, move on to the Bs. The Cs should be set aside completely (although sometimes I do these low-priority tasks as a short break from harder jobs).

The second model is from Stephen Covey's bestseller *The 7 Habits of Highly Effective People.* The Covey model is based on a crucial distinction between things that are urgent and those that are important. Urgency and importance may seem like the same thing, but they're not. Urgency merely reflects very short time frames, but it may involve trivial matters. Important tasks often involve long-term goals. Also, what may be urgent to someone else may not be urgent to you. If you feel you're constantly putting out fires or lurching from crisis to crisis, you're probably not making the distinction between "important" and "urgent" in your management of time.

> "Time is Nature's way of keeping everything from happening at once." Unknown

Dr. Covey uses a "Time Management Matrix" (see page 99) to illustrate his principle.

There are four quadrants. The top left is for tasks that are both urgent and important. Obviously, this is the place to start. The bottom right contains tasks that are neither urgent nor important. So why even bother doing them? These items should simply fall off the table.

The key question is which quadrant should be second. Dr. Covey advocates doing the important things, even if they're not urgent (the top right quadrant). In fact, if you deal with tasks *before* they are urgent, they'll never actually *become* urgent.

Time Management Matrix

	Urgent	Not Urgent
Important		
Not Important		

This is a key to good prioritization: you need to be more *proactive* and less reactive.

- Make a list of the tasks you intend to do over the next week.
- Make a To Do list for tomorrow. Beside each item put an A, B or C based on Lakein's criteria. (If you're undecided, ask yourself, "Is this important, urgent, both or neither?")
- Start your day with an A priority task. Once you've finished (or have made good progress), move on to the next item (another A or the top B task).
- As things come up during the day, pause before you jump into them. Ask yourself whether they're more important than what you're already working on.

David Posen, M.D.

Just as in a busy ER, your To Do list is not cast in stone. It's a constant re-juggling and balancing act between discipline and flexibility.

Delegating

Stop Multi-Tasking and Start Multi-Plexing

IMAGINE THIS SCENARIO: Phil Mickelson is playing in a golf tournament, and you're invited! You watch him tee off, after which he picks up his bag and walks down the fairway with his caddie, Jim MacKay, strolling beside him. He gets to his ball, pulls out an iron, hits the shot, replaces his divot and continues walking. On the green, he takes out his putter, removes the flag and putts out. Again carrying his own clubs, he proceeds to the next tee, washes off his ball, pulls out his driver and prepares to tee off again. Wouldn't it strike you as rather odd that the world's greatest golfer hires a caddie and then does all the work himself? Actually, it wouldn't just be odd—it'd be crazy! Yet this is what thousands of people do in the workplace every day. They hire support staff and then do the work themselves, often staying late to finish. There's something wrong with this picture.

There's an expression, "If you have a dog, why should *you* bark?" Delegation is an important skill, but most people don't do it very well. Scores of my patients have staff they can delegate to, but they still do too many things themselves and then wonder why they can't finish their work. Many people do two or three things at once (for example, reading their mail while talking on the phone) in order to "save time." But instead of multi-tasking, they should be "multi-plexing." This is a concept that occurred to me when one of my patients said, "I wish I could clone myself." I told him that if he trained his assistant properly it would be like duplicating himself. He was amazed at how well this worked.

> "Delegate everything but genius. Frank Sinatra didn't move pianos."
> Dan Sullivan, The Strategic Coach

There are four main reasons why people don't delegate:

1. They feel that no one else can do things exactly the way they'd like.

2. They have trouble giving up control.

3. They feel they don't have time to train someone to do the tasks.

4. They don't want to overburden others, especially those who are already over-loaded.

Let's go back to Phil Mickelson. I used to think that having a caddie was about luxury and privilege—something for rich folks. But really it's an arrangement to maximize efficiency, so that Phil can concentrate on his playing. Dan Sullivan mentors entrepreneurs at The Strategic Coach in Toronto. One of his teachings is "Delegate everything but genius." As he puts it, "Frank Sinatra didn't move pianos." It's wasteful for managers or self-employed professionals to be fielding phone calls, addressing envelopes or running errands. I was slow to learn this lesson, but having done so, I can personally attest to the tremendous results—less pressure on me and an increase in work output.

But aside from benefits to the *delegators*, there are also pluses for the delegates. In an efficient workplace, everybody should be doing all the tasks they're capable of and should be taught new skills to increase their capabilities. This isn't about overloading people or "buck passing." It's about utilizing their intelligence, skills and talents to the maximum level. The result is that workers feel valued, trusted and respected. They also feel stimulated, challenged, proud of the responsibility they've been given and validated by the contribution they can make. When done properly, delegating is a win-win. (When it's done badly, it can be unfair, exploitive or even abusive.)

In the army, they just ask for "volunteers." In life, it works differently.

Delegating is an important aspect of good time management—which, in turn, leads to improved work–life balance and less stress. It involves a trade-off: you get to make better use of your time in exchange for giving up some control. It also acknowledges that you can't do everything yourself. Delegates may not do tasks as well as you would do them—but they might surprise you and do them better!

Here are some delegating guidelines:

- Pick the right people to delegate to. Ask yourself, "Who could be doing this instead of me?"

- Give them clear instructions. Take the time to teach new skills.

- Confirm that they understand the assignment and when you want it completed.

- Stand back. Give them room to maneuver. Check in periodically, but don't hover.

- Be available to coach or give feedback.

- Hold them accountable for their work (quality and timeliness).

- Modify your expectations as required. Avoid perfectionism.

- Give praise—and always say "thank you."

This week, pick a task someone else could be doing that would free up your time.

Choose the most appropriate person to delegate to.

Be sensitive to his current workload—and help him to re-prioritize if necessary.

Take a few minutes to explain what you want and when you need it.

Get on with other work. Don't micromanage. Show your confidence in him.

David Posen, M.D.

The next time you see Phil Mickelson walking down the fairway with his caddie doing all the "heavy lifting," don't look at it as privilege. See it as an example of appropriate delegation that allows "Lefty" to display his legendary talent!

There's an Art to Conversation

ALK ABOUT A MISSED COMMUNICATION! Back when I was in my twenties, I was in a new relationship and we were spending a lot of time together on weekends. However, I'd been playing football on Sunday mornings since high school, and it was one of the highlights of my week. One Sunday, I decided to be a real prince and skip the game to spend time with my new romance. So, feeling virtuous, I announced my noble intention—although inwardly I felt a bit conflicted.

A week later, the truth came out. In a discussion resembling O. Henry's "The Gift of the Magi," I finally admitted I'd given up my football game to please her. Then she revealed that she'd been looking forward to a quiet morning of reading and had shelved her plans so as not to hurt my feelings. So here we were, two well-meaning people who, in trying to please each other, ended up pleasing no one. I learned two lessons that day: we needed to communicate better, and couples don't have to do everything together.

The consequences of *this* missed communication were minimal—and we even had a good laugh about of it. But some unstated messages have more serious effects, including tension, confusion and hurt feelings. For example: Party A doesn't invite Party B to a bridal shower. Party B feels slighted and offended. Party A later explains: "I was trying to spare you—from having to buy a gift and being bored out of your mind with all those strangers."

Every discussion has two parts: the content and the process.

Another problem in communication is *mixed* messages, where people may say one thing and do another or may just send out contradictory messages. Patients tell me about their performance appraisals. Some get lots of praise and high ratings, but are then told they won't be getting their bonus this year. Or the comments are glowing but their rating is "satisfactory." (They want to ask, "Are we talking about the same person here?") I once had a summer job in which my boss kept smiling and glad-handing me for two months, then gave me a lousy evaluation on the final day, when it was too late for me to do anything about it. You may know someone who blows hot and cold—one day you're her best friend, the next day she's too busy to talk to you. You don't know where you stand. If you feel confused or off balance with certain people, it may be because you're getting mixed signals from them.

Here are some thoughts on improving communication:

- **Distinguish between content and process.** Every discussion has two parts: the content, or subject matter, and the process, or dynamics, of the conversation. The content might be parenting issues, financial problems, social plans, home renovations or each other's behavior. The process might involve one person monopolizing the conversation (the other has to make a reservation to get a word in!), not paying attention while the other is talking, rambling and going off topic, asking a question and not waiting to hear the answer—or refuting the answer as soon as it's given.

    When people argue or get upset, they may think the conflict is over content when, in fact, it's often about process. People develop patterns of communication. Whatever the topic of conversation, their dynamics are remarkably similar. Start noticing people's communication style when you find it stressful to talk to them. Then point out the aspects that bother you.

- **Listen to the other person's "reality."** This takes discipline and an open mind, but you can learn a lot if you just listen to understand, not to judge. Be genuinely interested in hearing how the world looks to the other person. For example, if someone doesn't like crowds or big parties, don't say, "You're kidding—I love them!" Ask "Why is that hard for you? Help me to understand what that's like for you." And then listen to the answer.

> Communication is the currency of relationships—and we still don't do it very well.

- **Avoid "right/wrong, good/bad, win/lose" conversations.** A discussion is not a debate in which the winner gets a trophy. It should be an honest exchange of ideas and information, a sharing of feelings or an attempt to solve a problem. If you stop trying to score points, you can learn a lot more about each other and have a better conversation. This leads to decreased tension, improved relationships and, possibly, more intimacy and closeness.

- **Keep it simple—and brief.** Sometimes less is more. Avoid rambling and lecturing. This is especially true with kids: if it's not short and sweet, they tune out.

- **Listening is as important as talking**—probably more so. But really listen; don't just be thinking about what you are going to say next or look for an opening to jump in. And if people take a moment to answer a question, be patient. Don't start talking over their thinking time.

- **Listen to understand and empathize, not to problem solve.** My wife taught me this valuable lesson. I was a family doctor at the time. Patients brought me their problems and expected me to solve them. I got used to the role of "fixer." But that's not what my wife wanted from me. Sometimes people just want to be heard. They're not looking for answers or solutions. They don't want your brilliant advice—especially when it's unsolicited! They just want you to listen and to care.

- **Choose when and where to talk.** Timing is important in communication. Don't try to engage someone when they're tired or busy. Some people want to get into heavy conversations at bedtime. Or they bring up a contentious issue as the other person is leaving for work. Be sensitive to the other person's preferences if you want a receptive listener. It helps to arrange a time or ask "When would be a good time for you?"

Identify one person you find stressful to talk to.

See if you can pinpoint what it is you find frustrating or off-putting.

Think about how you might prevent or deal with that problem.

Consider discussing it with him—openly and constructively.

Start to be aware of your own communication style and how it can be improved.

David Posen, M.D.

Missed messages, mixed messages, monopolizing and motor-mouthing are all stressful. But sometimes the biggest problem is lack of communication—when people don't talk to each other at all!

The Other Side of Progress

I WAS INVITED TO GIVE A WORKSHOP for a group of high-powered executives. It was held at a small lakeside resort on a sunny day in June—an idyllic setting for talking about work–life balance and values. At the mid-morning break, I noticed three group members chatting out on the driveway. But they weren't talking to one another. Each had a phone against his ear, presumably talking about business. Well, I thought, maybe some things can't wait. But then I looked out the lakeside window at another group on the deck. Despite the lovely view, they also had BlackBerries and cellphones stuck to their ears, and each was preoccupied with a seemingly important conversation. What's wrong with this picture? We were gathered for a peaceful retreat on a beautiful lake to get some perspective on our lives—and these guys were trying to fit business into the cracks!

This is not an isolated incident. At workshops I watch people stampede to pay phones instead of enjoying those tasty snacks. I've often asked people to turn off their laptops during seminar breaks. They reply that if they don't constantly pick up their messages, they'll have a hundred e-mails to deal with by the end of the day.

We live in a wired world. It's a mixed blessing. I remember the breakthrough when doctors got pagers. They allowed us to be out and about when we were on call instead of being tied to a telephone. What freedom! However, in today's world, smartphones, cell phones, voice mail and e-mail have created an electronic leash instead of liberation. As David Brooks put it in a *Newsweek* article, "Never being out of touch means never being able to get away."

"Never being out of touch means never being able to get away."

And this isn't the only kind of communication aggravation. We've all been on trains and buses where one insensitive passenger with a cell phone and a loud voice can infuriate dozens of travelers who want only to read or sleep. We also get to learn far more about the extrovert (make that exhibitionist) than any of us wanted to know.

Here's another scenario. I recently called the help line for one of my office techno-gizmos that was on the fritz. I was then led through a maze of voice-mail menus the likes of which I'd never encountered before. They were so multi-layered you needed to draw flow diagrams to keep track of all the options. The meta-message it conveyed was, "We've already made the sale. We're not interested in your problem. Go away!" After three rounds of this charade, I hung up, called the dealer from whom I'd bought the equipment and said, "I'd like you to handle this. Your supplier doesn't seem to be very customer-focused."

Then there's the steady stream of misdirected faxes I receive that are meant for a professional office in town with a fax number similar to mine. This leads to questions of "fax etiquette." Do I ignore them (and risk being a bad citizen), resend them to the proper number (which takes time—some of these documents are ten to twenty pages long), call the senders (or intended recipients) to tell them their message went astray? And who should pay for all the paper and ink these unwanted faxes consume? Unsolicited marketing faxes are another plague, adding to *your* overhead costs while the advertiser incurs no expense at all. Great racket—no wonder there's so much of it.

Then there's the "hurry-up" factor. A lawyer told me: "I used to get letters asking for an opinion. I'd think about it and mail back a reply. Now I get an e-mail asking for a response by 2:00 today. Then I receive a phone call an hour later, asking, 'Did you get my e-mail? What do you think?'" This acceleration of expected turnaround is not only stressful, but often precludes time for reflection. We're expected to react rather than respond. And unless we do something about it, it's only going to get worse.

> First these toys were novel, then they became indispensable, and now they're running our lives.

Finally, my pet peeve: call waiting—which I label "call aggravating." I understand the need for businesses to answer each call, which sometimes means putting people on hold. But residential phones where each incoming call beeps a signal to interrupt? Persistently? Every time a phone partner says, "Oh, just a second, let me get this call," I feel like they're really saying," Hold on a sec—this call might be more important than you." What a great technological invention! How did we ever get along without it? (I know many people disagree with me on this one—including my siblings!)

Did I mention spam e-mails that take several minutes to download and delete? Or those error messages that tell you that you can't connect with your Internet server—just as you're tidying up to go on vacation? These are some of the joyous wired-world experiences that I call Communication Aggravation. It's time to tame this monster that's taking over our lives.

Dealing with Information Overload and Technostress

Who's the Master and Who's the Servant?

O DOUBT ABOUT IT. Advanced technology is here to stay. And it's invaded every part of our lives. But for every convenience there's a hassle. Talk about a mixed blessing! We have to get a handle on this: either we learn to use these gadgets, or they'll end up using us. Here are some suggestions:

GENERAL PRINCIPLES

1. Decide what technology you want to use and how you want to use it. You don't need every gadget just because it's available. I choose not to carry a pager, electronic organizer or laptop. I only recently got a cell phone—but I give the number to very few people. I have caller ID and take calls selectively during high-concentration work. I don't have a fax machine at home. These choices suit my business practice and lifestyle. Choose what works for you.

2. Tell people your favored method of communication. I prefer telephone first, e-mail second and fax third. I inform people that I check my e-mail only twice a day, so, to reach me quickly, telephone is best. My wife and I ask people not call us after 10:00 p.m.

3. Treat people the way *you* want to be treated. Don't spam others if you don't like them spamming you. Don't use your cell phone like a megaphone in public places.

> My two favorite residential phone messages that cut to the chase are "Speak at the beep" and "You know what to do."

4. Be selective about whom you give your cell phone number and e-mail address to.

VOICE MAIL

Receiving calls

1. Keep your recorded message short. Identify your name or company and invite a message. You can say "I'm sorry I missed your call," but don't list a bunch of reasons why you're not available. It doesn't matter if you're on another line, in a meeting, out for lunch, taking a walk or in the bathroom—the point is you're not available. My two favorite residential phone messages that cut to the chase are "Speak at the beep" and "You know what to do."

2. Tell callers if your machine has a time limit, so they don't get cut off in mid-sentence.

3. If you require a long message, use a bypass system that allows callers to get right to the "record" tone.

4. Avoid clichés—everyone's busy. I especially dislike "Your call is important to us," usually used by companies that never answer with a live voice.

5. If you're out, tell callers when you'll be picking up messages and calling back.

6. If you're away, program your phone to go into voice mail after one ring.

7. When you're involved in high-concentration tasks, avoid the temptation to answer the phone. It's a discipline—you may break out in a cold sweat—but it will protect your most productive time.

Leaving messages for others

1. Be brief. Anticipate a recorded greeting and plan your message in advance. Most of us don't think quickly enough to leave a concise message without this kind of planning.

2. State the purpose of your call and the best time to call you back.

3. Repeat your name and phone number at the end of your message (and say your number s-l-o-w-l-y).

4. Leave only one message—even if you call back two or three times.

FAX

1. Don't send unsolicited marketing faxes.

2. If you ignore #1, at least indicate how recipients can get off your mailing list.

3. Ask if people require a cover sheet and tell them if you don't need one. It saves a lot of time, ink and paper.

4. Be respectful of privacy. Don't send highly confidential information by fax. Unopened or misdirected letters are sealed, but faxes are open to anyone and may lie around for days.

> "Never let a computer know you're in a hurry."
>
> Unknown

E-MAIL

1. Check e-mail only once or twice a day. It's a tempting toy, but a sinkhole for time and energy.

2. Don't open your e-mail first thing in the morning if you're a morning person. You'll end up giving away your best thirty to sixty minutes each day, when you're freshest and most productive.

3. Turn off the sound on your computer that signals the arrival of each new e-mail.

4. Don't respond to messages unless you have to. Your quick "Thanks Bernie— have a great weekend," is just one more message for him to download, open, read and delete. It can be a greater courtesy not to reply.

5. Keep your messages short—it saves time for everyone.

6. If you're sending the same message to multiple people, use the "blind cc" option so the recipients see only their own name. I once received a four-line message that was preceded by sixteen lines of e-mail addresses.

7. Use high- or highest-priority designations only when you really mean it. I once got a message marked "highest priority" only to find a solicitation for a charitable donation.

8. Get your name taken off as many e-mail lists as possible. This includes joke lists—unless the jokes are really funny.

9. Use filtering programs if you're inundated with unwanted e-mails.

10. Be your own filtering system. Before you press Send, ask yourself if the message really needs to be sent at all.

Communication is a great thing. Over communication is a blight. Use your toys wisely—and encourage others to do the same.

• List all the technology tools you currently use (voice mail, e-mail, fax, cell phone, laptop, electronic calendar, etc.)

• Evaluate each on a scale of 1 to10 regarding
  — amount of use
  — ease of use
  — overall benefit
  — overall hassle

• Decide which ones serve you best and whether you can drop one or two (without breaking them!)

• Identify ways to streamline the way you use each gadget—to benefit yourself and others.

• Over the next week, implement the improvements you've just listed.

David Posen, M.D.

Handling Home Chores
It's a House, Not a Museum

O SCAR MADISON HAD IT MADE. In the Neil Simon play *The Odd Couple*, Oscar was a sportswriter slob who lived with his nit-picking, fuss-budget friend Felix Unger, a neat freak. Because Oscar didn't mind mess and chaos, he was off the hook for doing home chores. Felix, however, seemed to make it his life's work to pick up after Oscar and keep their Manhattan apartment looking clean and orderly. Despite his complaining and exasperation, Felix still did all the work!

In the work–life balancing act, home chores are the second biggest problem after hours spent at a paid job. Author Arlie Hochschild calls this the Second Shift. This problem still affects women more than men, although the gender gap is closing as men get more involved on the home front.

The best way to handle home chores is to share the load. Note that there's a difference between **helping** and **sharing**. When you ask someone to help, you are implying that this is *your* job, but you would like their assistance. When you ask them to share the load, the message is: "We all live here and there's work required to keep the house in order. It is no more *my* job than anyone else's. We all need to pitch in until it's done."

It's also important to distinguish between **equal** and **equitable** sharing. Equal sharing means that everybody is doing the same amount. An equitable division of labor is one that is acceptable to everybody even if the load is not shared equally. For example, one person might do the heavy yard work, and less of the lighter inside work. Or someone who doesn't like cooking might agree to do kitchen cleanups plus laundry in exchange for chef duty. Someone who has a very busy schedule or health problems might do less work but, relative to time constraints and physical ability, would still shoulder an acceptable amount of the load. The main criterion of equitable sharing is fairness:

> We all live here and there's work required to keep the house in order. We all need to pitch in until it's done.

everyone feels comfortable with the arrangement and no one feels taken advantage of or taken for granted.

Good communication is essential to effective teamwork. After years as a stay-at-home mom, one of my patients decided to take a part-time job. Not surprisingly, her family had gotten used to her doing almost all of the home chores. She called a meeting with her husband and children, told them her plans and requested their support. Then she laid it on the line: some things would have to change around the house if she was going to handle this additional role. She stated her expectations that the family would take more responsibility in meal preparation (including school lunches), kitchen cleanups, making beds, vacuuming and laundry. Her family didn't cheer with excitement, but they did agree they'd had it pretty easy and it was only fair that they now share the load. The successful formula here was Communication, Consideration and Cooperation.

Don't take better care of your house than you do of yourself.

Here are some timely tips:

- **Delegate to family members.** Even young children should be included. Train and coach as required.

- **Hire help.** If your funds allow, pay someone for housecleaning, grass cutting, snow shoveling, and so on.

- **Do some chores together.** Clean up your basement, garden or garage as a family. The work goes faster, it's more fun and it promotes togetherness.

- **Let some things go.** Do you really have to iron your sheets? Beds don't have to be made *every* morning—especially if you're in a hurry. If you're pressed for time, buy a cake when friends come over instead of baking your own. Avoid unnecessary make-work projects.

- **Do some things less often.** Wear clothes a little longer—or buy extra underwear, socks and towels to avoid frequent laundering.

- **Find shortcuts.** Fitted sheets and duvets were a big breakthrough in my life because they simplified bed making. One of my patients was thrilled to discover she could let dishes dry in a rack instead of using time and a towel.

- **Buy labor-saving appliances.** Dishwashers and microwaves are good investments. We bought a community snow-blower with four neighbors.

- **Cook extra servings and freeze for later use.** Cook in quantity: toss large salads twice a week, double your lasagna recipe. Simplify meal preparation.

- **Maintain realistic expectations.** When all else fails, lower your standards. Your house doesn't have to look like it's on permanent display. You don't have to shine the kitchen floor. Realistic expectations are especially important if you have young children. My wife and I got pretty good at stepping over piles of toys rather than picking up at every turn. The house was never a mess, it was just lived in.

- **Consider downsizing.** This is a more dramatic solution, but fewer rooms (and less furniture) means less hassle and more time for you.

R̸ₓ   This week, keep track, in writing, of the time you spend on home chores.

Pick one task that each family member can take on as their own. Help them get started.

Pick one chore that you can hire out. Find an appropriate person, such as a student.

Find one task that can be shortened, eliminated or done less frequently.

Identify one appliance that would save you time. Buy it or start to save for its purchase.

David Posen, M.D.

Felix Unger could have managed things better and saved himself a lot of hassle. But then the play would have closed in Albany!

Procrastination

Learning the Art of "Doing it Now"

ONFESSION: TWO YEARS AGO I bought a book about procrastination—but I never got around to reading it. Not that this was anything new. My favorite time was always the eleventh hour.

Here's how I almost missed going to med school: I was working at a summer camp when I realized that the deadline for applying to pre med was only days away. The application form was about eight pages long. No wonder I'd been putting it off for months! Suddenly, it was panic time. There I was, sitting on my bunk filling out pages of autobiographical information and answering questions such as "Why do you want to be a doctor?" (This was especially challenging for me to answer because I really wanted to be a teacher.) After finishing the last page, I saw that they required a photograph. "Terrific," I thought, "Now I'm really cooked!" Not only did I not have one, but there was no time to get one from home. Suddenly I had a brain wave: one of my campers had a Polaroid camera (they were new at the time—and no, I'm not ninety). He agreed to take my picture. Wearing my only dress clothes, I got all gussied up on this sweltering summer day, stood against the cabin door and had Jeff snap off a photo. From the waist up, I looked very respectable; from the waist down I was in shorts and bare feet. We cropped the picture, slapped it on the application and fired it off to the University of Toronto.

> One way to make jobs less intimidating is to break them down into smaller parts.

But my procrastination didn't end there. When I was actually accepted for med school, I put off phoning in to accept my place in the class. After several days of reminding me, my *brother* phoned the university to say that I'd be there.

Procrastination is a common human behavior, but a very costly one. Aside from the stress of last-minute panic, there are other consequences. One of my patients put off sending in his expense accounts and receipts for months, which meant that money that could have been in his bank account stayed in the company's account instead. People who are late filing their income tax pay hefty penalties, plus interest on the unpaid taxes. Then there's the embarrassment of running into someone who sent you a beautiful wedding gift six months earlier, to whom you never got around to writing a thank-you note. Is it worth it to delay getting your car repaired for so long that the warranty runs out? Or to put off filling up your car until you run out of gas on the highway? Or to wait so long to order theater tickets that they're sold out by the time you phone?

Why do people procrastinate? The list is long. Which ones apply to you?

- disorganization

- a desire to avoid unpleasant tasks

- fear of failure

- conversely, fear of success and the implications it might have for your life

- a feeling that the project is so overwhelming you don't know where to start

- perfectionism (you don't want to do it unless, and until, you can do it perfectly)

- lack of confidence and negative self-talk

- fear of change

- fear of rejection (job-hunters and salespeople confront this continually)

- the task looks too hard and time consuming

- you don't have the supplies or resources needed to do the job

There are a host of other excuses. Note, though, that, at times, procrastination serves a valuable purpose: your inner voice may be saying, "I really don't want to do this at all—ever."

> "Emmett's Law: The dread of doing a task uses up more time and energy than doing the task itself."
> Rita Emmett

One way to make jobs less intimidating is to break them down into smaller parts. Big projects look daunting; smaller ones feel easier. This is sometimes called the "Swiss cheese" method—it's like taking small bites out of a big piece of cheese rather than trying to eat it all at once.

Make a list of the steps needed to complete the task you're putting off. List all the supplies and equipment you'll need. Assemble the necessary resources. Then work on one step at a time as if each is a task in itself. And don't forget to reward yourself at the end of each stage.

Make a list of all the things you've been putting off. Make it a long list.

Beside each item, write down why you've been delaying. Be honest. Then, see if there are common themes.

Pick one item on the list to address this week (writing a report, cleaning up your closet, organizing a party).

Choose a time this week to do it. Assemble the things you'll need for the job.

Set a kitchen timer for one hour. Just get started—no interruptions, no breaks, no distractions.

David Posen, M.D.

By the way, I finally read the book *The Procrastinator's Handbook* by Rita Emmett. It was terrific. I should have done it sooner!

Do You Really Need All That Stuff?

ERE'S A GUTSY WAY to test your marriage. A couple was moving house and had decided to purge their wardrobes. Each of them struggled over which clothes to throw out. Progress was minimal and frustration high.

Editorial comments and playful digs were made about each other's selections: "You never wear that. Why are you keeping it?" and "That was even out of style when you bought it!" Finally, they came up with a creative idea. They traded places. Each started to prune the other's pile of clothes. This led to some interesting dynamics: if one got too ruthless, they knew the other would do the same. So a level of fairness and restraint quickly set in. They helped each other make sensible and necessary choices they weren't able to make on their own. It was also a good test of their relationship—which, fortunately, survived.

Whether it's clothes, books, gadgets, tools, party hats or notes from high school, clutter creates many problems. It encroaches on usable space in your home and office. It creates confusion and inefficiency. It can spawn fire hazards or breeding grounds for mold and vermin. When things are hard to find, that leads to stress. Remember the last time you needed something urgently and had to plow through piles of stuff in a panicked search for the elusive item? (Winter boots on the morning of the first snowstorm come to mind.) Clutter leads to poor organization and can even become overwhelming.

I can personally attest to the benefits of decluttering. After a massive office cleanup years ago, I could see the top of my desk again. It was great! I felt a sense

> Have a place for everything and put everything in its place.

of lightness and relief. I felt energized. Decluttering makes you feel more organized and in control. And every so often you come across some lost treasure you'd thought had vanished forever. Then there's the pleasure of giving things away to people you know will appreciate them. If you have enough good stuff, you can hold a garage sale—a thoroughly purging exercise based on the premise that one person's garbage is another person's gold (well, okay, silver or bronze).

Here are some decluttering strategies:

1. Work out a system for large areas (if you're cleaning a room, start with one corner).

2. Have a reality check. Don't keep something just because you "might need it some day." And stop pretending that some day you're going to get that banjo fixed and learn to play it again.

3. Be ruthless. If you find your motivation waning, ask someone to help you—or take a break and return with a fresh perspective.

4. Have a place for everything and put everything in its place.

5. Get boxes, baskets or storage bins to put similar items in and label them clearly.

6. Develop a storage system. Tools should be stored together; photos should all be in albums or boxes; winter hats, scarves and mitts should all be in one place; luggage, totes and athletic bags should have their own area; and so on. Our family has a "birthday bag" for streamers, signs, candles and paper plates.

7. Develop a recycling system. My wife put a plastic shelving unit in our main floor utility closet. We place cans and bottles on top, plastic bags on the next level, newspapers and magazines on the third shelf, cardboard next, and corrugated cardboard on the bottom. When blue box day comes, it takes mere minutes to get everything out to the curb because it's been stored in an organized way for the preceding two weeks.

> "You can't have everything.
> Where would you put it?"
> Stephen Wright

8. Put your unwanted items in three separate containers: one for trash, one to give away to specific individuals, one for donations to local charities.

9. Consider having a garage sale (on your own or with neighbors). Used clothes can be sold on consignment at some stores; used books might be bought by second-hand bookstores.

10. Once you've decluttered an area, guard against reaccumulating another load of stuff. Be more mindful in the things you buy and accept from others.

Select one area of your home or office—a drawer, a cupboard or an entire room—that's become a clutter nightmare.

Pick a time this week to clean up the messy space, or at least to get a good start. Give yourself at least an hour.

Take everything out and sort it into three piles: keepers, obvious discards and items you're not sure about.

Selectively put back the "keepers." Organize a storage system to keep things orderly.

Scrutinize the "not sure" items and ask yourself honestly when was the last time you used them. If they're damaged, haven't been worn or used in the last two years, or you don't enjoy them anymore, out they go.

Decide whether to throw your discards in the garbage or give them away.

David Posen, M.D.

Incidentally, the wardrobe-pruning couple I described are still together—and extremely well-dressed—more than thirty years later.

We're Still Drowning in Paper

HATEVER HAPPENED TO BILL GATES'S notion of the paperless office? A few years ago, I did a major paper purge of my office. Today, I'm digging out again as if a blizzard had hit while I wasn't looking. Junk mail, faxes, reports, research articles and information bulletins abound. I get a slew of magazines and journals that I never ordered, but that have interesting information in them. Catalogs and manuals get thicker every year. Some monthly magazines are as fat as phone books. Rules and regulations about how long to keep documents make me reluctant to pitch anything that looks halfway important. What's a guy to do?

I'm not alone. A recent newspaper squib noted that the use of paper has increased by 40% since the advent of fax machines, computers and e-mail. Most of us are drowning in paper. One store generates a full-page receipt when I buy batteries for $4.95. This creates stress, frustration and a loss of control—not to mention the occasional panic when you can't find important documents. Much has been written about taming this beast—also, of course, on paper!

How do we bail ourselves out? For starters, we need time, a filing system, a steely resolve and discipline! The decluttering process involves three stages:

Stage 1: Sorting and purging the accumulated junk

Pick an area that's become a paper disaster. Gather up all the loose paper (newspapers, magazines, mail, invoices, invitations, correspondence, etc.) into one pile. Now get four containers (baskets or small boxes will do) and sort into four groups: to act on, to file, to read and to pitch (your trash can is the most important container!).

Every piece of paper represents a decision you've put off in the past.

Stage 1 has two purposes: purging the junk and dividing the rest for action and storage. Don't get bogged down or start reading stuff. Just put each piece of paper into one of the four boxes. You'll have to make some tough choices. Every piece of paper represents a decision you've put off in the past. You may break into a cold sweat at the thought of parting with things. Stay with it! Toss anything that's out of date. If you have several related articles, just save one or two. With magazines and journals, rip out and staple the articles you want to read, then chuck the rest of the magazine.

Stage 2: Organizing and storing what you decide to keep

a) Go through the "to act on" container. Separate bills that have to be paid or time-sensitive correspondence. Put these in their own folder or basket for immediate attention.

b) Now for the "to file" container. Get a filing cabinet with at least two drawers— preferably ones that take hanging files. Buy a set of alphabetical dividers and some file folders. Then go through your pile one sheet at a time and sort into categories: receipts, insurance, manuals, warranties, photos, health documents, financial records, tax information, cards, letters, etc. Create a file for each category and label it. Don't keep everything. Be selective. According to organization guru Stephanie Culp, 80% of what you file will never be looked at again.

   Another organizing expert, Barbara Hemphill, suggests asking yourself these questions to guide your decision making:

   1. Did I ask for this information?

   2. Is this the only place the information is available?

   3. Is the information recent enough to be useful?

   4. Can I identify specific circumstances when I would want this information?

   5. Are there are any tax or legal implications?

   6. What's the worst possible thing that could happen if I didn't have this piece of paper?

c) Next comes the "to read" pile. If you're like me, you've saved interesting articles from magazines or stuff sent to you by friends. You envision sitting outside on a summer afternoon and sifting through this fascinating material. But when that time arrives, you'll probably want to read the new book you just bought or the up-to-date article that arrived in today's mail. Experts will tell you to stop pretending you're going to read this stuff someday. It ain't gonna happen. Most of this material you can heave now.

File your "keepers" in labeled folders (health, world events, financial advice, etc.). Try this reality check: write the date on each file, then go through it in three months and see what you've actually read. After six months, it's bye-bye time!

> "The average worker spends 150 hours per year looking for information."
>
> Barbara Hemphill

When you're done, you'll feel a lot lighter, more organized, more in control and maybe even a tad smug (it's well deserved). And you'll be able to find things in a nano-second.

Stage 3: Controlling the future inflow of paper and making the process ongoing

This requires time—paper doesn't sort itself. You need to purge your files periodically. But mostly you need to control the inflow of paper. I've dropped one magazine subscription in each of the last three years. I rarely buy magazines, newspapers or books unless I'm likely to read them soon. (Why pay for more clutter?) Be careful about what you print out from the Internet. Open your mail beside the garbage pail.

- Set aside two to three hours in the next week to do a paper purge.
- Pick an area to work on: your office, your desk, even one drawer or cupboard.
- Get your four containers ready—including a big trash can or, better yet, a recycling bin.
- Have your supplies—filing cabinet, file folders, labeling pens—ready.
- Get started.

David Posen, M.D.

Next month I'm planning another major cleanup. Maybe I should invite Bill Gates over to give me a hand!

Money and Stress

It's Time to Face the Music

MY FRIEND DAVE CALLED it the Law of Rotating Bankruptcy. Here's how it works. You're short of money, so you borrow from Friend A. Once he lends you the money, you're flush but he's a bit thin. At some point, he gets tapped out and turns to Friend B for a short-term loan. Now he's okay again, but Friend B is strapped for funds. You get a paycheck and pay off Friend A, who's now in the money. But only briefly. He then pays off Friend B, and so it goes. This is how a lot of us got through our school years. We took turns having money and *not* having money.

The problem is that some people keep living that way, always close to the line. They continually borrow from Peter to pay Paul. Only now their "friends" are banks and credit cards. The cost is not only high interest rates, but also high stress.

Financial pressures and worries are big stressors in today's world. Most people are constantly struggling to stay afloat. I've seen two bumper stickers that reflect this problem: "Can I pay off my MasterCard with my Visa?" and "I can't be overdrawn—I still have checks left!"

But a shortage of funds is not the only way money and stress are related. Another issue is how money is used. Many couples argue because one wants to save while the other wants to spend ("I'm not here for a long time; I'm here for a good time!"). This is a conflict in *values*. Couples also have different *priorities*: one may want to redo the basement, while the other wants to take a trip—and they can't afford both. The result is tension and frustration.

> When people talk about money, it's never about money.

Then there's the stress attached to simply *getting* more money—working long hours, taking a second job—the endless and futile "earn and spend cycle." Many people stay in jobs they hate until their pension is fully vested or they get a good severance package.

125

People who *have* money get financial headaches too, especially when the stock markets plunge. These people fret over how to invest and who to turn to for advice. (I once heard this definition of a financial advisor: a person you give your money to until there's none left). They also put themselves into daily fits watching the stock market roller-coaster.

People do interesting things when it comes to money. Consider planned spending versus *impulsive* spending. Guess which uses up the most dough? Window shopping is one thing, but if you actually walk into the store, I'm betting you'll buy something you don't need.

Then there's the "who pays for what" game. When I was growing up, boys paid for *everything* when they took girls on dates. I'd go out on a Saturday night with $10 to pay for a movie and snacks; my twin sister would happily sail out with her date carrying a single dime (in case she had to make a phone call).

And what about restaurant etiquette? Four people go out for a meal. Three have steaks with wine, the fourth has soup and salad. Should they split the bill four ways? The light eater feels stressed if he subsidizes his friends—but speaking up is *also* stressful.

There's also the "power trip" game: theatrics about who's going to pick up the check. One guy never even offers, while others fight over who's going to be a sport (or show-off) and treat the other three.

Let's not forget the "control" game, in which one person controls the purse strings and very stringently doles out bits of money to a partner, who has to justify every purchase and must ask permission to buy a $5 magazine.

Money and stress: there are myriad connections. And, in at least one, money can actually be a stress *reliever*. Many people buy a new item of clothing or a new gadget when they're stressed out, to give themselves a lift. It's called "Retail Therapy"!

"The safest way to double your money is to fold it over once and put it in your pocket."

I've learned two interesting things from my patients. One is that money means different things to different people. A friend of mine puts it this way: "When people talk about money, it's never about *money*." It's about security, freedom, luxury, power and status, fairness, responsibility, trust—and values! It might mean still other things to you.

The other observation is that people's financial stress is not related to the *amount* of money they have. I've seen people anguish over money whether they have a little or a lot. Conversely, it's not unusual to hear patients say, "My financial situation is actually a little worse now than it was six months ago, but I'm less stressed about it."

SUGGESTIONS FOR MANAGING YOUR MONEY

1. **Distinguish "wants" from "needs."** Be mindful of how you spend your money. Food, shelter and basic clothing are needs. All other choices are *wants*.

2. **Discipline your spending.** When you go to the mall, decide what you need, buy it and leave. This will save time as well as money. Browsing leads to impulse spending—those merchandisers are smarter than you are!

3. **Pay yourself first.** Take 10% of your paycheck and immediately put it into savings. Don't let it even touch your fingers. You'll notice two things: 1) it starts to add up quickly, and 2) if you park it before you ever see it, you don't miss it.

4. **Pay off debt as quickly as possible.** As my father taught me, "interest will kill you." Pay off high-interest debts first (especially credit cards). Next, get rid of debt that's not tax-deductible. Carry only one or two credit cards—cut up all others. Pay off your credit card balance in full each month. Otherwise, pay cash.

5. **Track your spending** for a few months to see where your money's going. Write down everything you spend. You may be shocked to see that your daily soup and sandwich at lunch costs $35 a week and extra roaming or data charges on your smartphone can creep up on you. It all adds up.

6. **Live within your means**—based on your *after*-tax (net) income.

7. **If you're having problems managing your money, seek professional help.** Most communities have consumer credit counseling services available.

R℞ . Sit down this week and write out a financial statement. Record your assets (investments, savings, home and car values, etc.) and liabilities (loans, mortgage, credit card debt).

. Calculate your monthly expenses: fixed (mortgage or rent, phone, utilities, insurance) and variable (groceries, gas, clothes, haircuts, etc.). Then compare your monthly outflow with your monthly income. Are you spending more than you're earning?

. Write down everything you spend over the next week and get into the habit of tracking where your money goes.

. Pick one area of discretionary spending to stop (your morning donut and coffee, for example).

. Decide which loan or debt to pay off first. Make even a token payment this week.

David Posen, M.D.

It's time to take control of your money and be mindful of how you use it. Then the Law of Rotating Bankruptcy will no longer apply to you.

Trouble Making Decisions
Ask Your Friends, Flip a Coin—or Read This

A FRIEND OF MINE TELLS A STORY about the time she and I went shopping in Los Angeles to find me a new bathing suit. We went to a couple of stores and looked at a million bathing suits. I just couldn't decide. There was so much to choose from—bathing trunks in every style and color imaginable. To her credit, my friend was amazingly tolerant and patient. Later I realized how close she must have been to tearing her hair out—or mine. You'd have thought I was buying a beach house, not beach wear!

In retrospect, I think there were two problems: there were far too many choices, and nothing really felt suitable (pardon the pun). Stuck with what felt like a bunch of second choices, I simply couldn't make up my mind.

Ironically, I made the decision to change careers within days, and I bought my last car within hours of test-driving it. There are times when we just know the decision is right. At other times (often with more trivial choices), we can dither endlessly.

Difficulty making decisions is a symptom of stress, but can also be a *source* of stress. Uncertainty leads to feelings of insecurity, confusion and loss of control. Over my years as a physician, I've helped patients struggle with big and difficult decisions (leaving a marriage, quitting a job, selling a house). While I can't decide for them, I can help them with the process, and help them live with whatever decision they make. Here are some approaches I've found helpful:

> Ask what's the best and worst that can happen. Then weigh upside benefits versus downside risks.

1. List all the options you can think of.

Don't edit yourself at this stage—just make the most complete list you can. For example, in a severe marriage conflict, the options aren't simply to stay or leave. They include:

a) Staying put and accepting the status quo

b) Staying together but working on the marriage and trying to make it better

c) Staying in the marriage and getting professional counseling

d) Staying in the marriage, but living separate lives

e) Trial separation (with or without professional counseling)

f) Permanent separation

g) Divorce

    After you've listed your options, eliminate those that are unacceptable to you. Then number the remaining items in order of preference. Finally, decide which option to pursue. Then formulate a plan of action.

2. Use a "Ben Franklin balance sheet."

I've used this helpful technique for years with patients and in my own life. Take an issue you're struggling with and list all the pros and cons of each option. We had a summer cottage that we had doubts about (especially the three-hour drive). One day we discussed selling it. We set up a grid sheet with four quadrants as shown below.

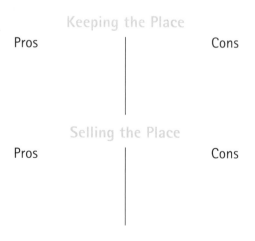

Keeping the Place

Pros | Cons

Selling the Place

Pros | Cons

Then we listed all the pros and cons we could think of. You might expect that all the pros for Keeping the Place would simply be repeated in the cons of Selling the Place. But by shifting your perspective from "staying" to "leaving," you actually generate different ideas. This exercise helped us explore the issue fully, and the decision became clearer.

Not all the factors will be of equal importance. Deal with this by highlighting the most significant points or by using a rating scale.

Even when the balance sheet doesn't give you a clear answer, it helps to clarify the issues. In this sense, the process can be as important as the final decision.

3. Ask what's the best and worst that can happen. Then weigh upside benefits versus downside risks.

A friend called me with a hot investment tip: a secure second mortgage paying 4% higher than current rates. I bounced it off my brother, who is very wise in these matters. He asked two questions: "If it's so secure, why are they paying a 4% premium?" and "How much are you planning to invest?" I said, "$5,000." He did the math: "The extra 4% would increase your return by only $200 a year (your potential upside benefit). But your downside risk is that you could lose the whole $5,000. I wouldn't touch it." Put in those terms, the decision was easy.

> "When you come to a fork in the road, take it."
> Yogi Berra

4. Don't look for the perfect decision.

A patient was struggling with a difficult decision. We listed all her options and every one of them had serious drawbacks. Finally I suggested we change our perspective: "Let's stop looking for a good solution—there isn't one. Just pick the one that's least bad."

5. Imagine you've already made the decision and notice how you feel.

One of my patients was struggling with a decision. Finally, I said, "It sounds like a tie to me. Why don't we just flip a coin?" She said, "Okay." As soon as she saw that it was tails, her face dropped. "Do you want to go two out of three?"

I asked. She quickly said, "Yeah." In that moment, she realized that her reaction was an indication of her real preference.

6. Use the 80/20 rule.

In today's fast-moving business world, decisions have to be made quickly, often without all the relevant information. A rough rule of thumb is that, if you have 80% of the information you need, you've got enough to make the decision.

- Pick one area of indecision you're struggling with right now.
- List all the possible options you can think of.
- Rank your choices in order of preference.
- Choose your top pick and create a game plan for acting on it.
- If you're still not sure, pick your top two options and run them through the Ben Franklin balance sheet.

David Posen, M.D.

And the next time you're shopping for a bathing suit and don't see anything you like, leave the store. And always take your fashion advisor with you!

Long-Distance Worrying

Life Has Enough Challenges—Don't Start Early on New Ones

I SAW A PATIENT THIS MORNING with a very common problem. She woke up twice in the night worrying about problems at work. And while some of the issues were current, many were more general and related to things that won't happen for a long time, if at all.

Worrying is both a cause and a symptom of stress. It's also a terrible drain on time and energy. Some worrying is normal and inevitable—such as when your teenager is still out two hours after curfew. But some people worry weeks or months in advance. It's as if they're trying to get a head start so they can be miserable for as long as possible. This is a real time waster—especially since most of the things we worry about never come to pass. I call it "long-distance worrying." One of my patients called it "borrowing trouble from the future."

Some people believe that worrying wards off trouble. One of my patients calls it "preventive worrying." His theory is that if he worries about something, it won't happen. Since it's impossible to prove, this can be a difficult notion to dispel. It's like the story of the guy who's snapping his fingers all the time. Somebody asks him, "Why are you doing that?"

"To keep the elephants away."

"There are no elephants within 5,000 miles of here."

"See, it works!"

> "A day of worry is more exhausting than a week of work." Unknown

During the 1990s, a lot of worrying was about job security in an era of downsizing, restructuring and mergers. People became hypersensitive to every nuance in the workplace. Any directive or off-hand remark was seen as a potential tip-off about some change in company policy. I learned to take a different approach to these matters. Whenever there were rumors of new government policy regarding doctors, I chose to take a "wait and see" approach and not get caught up in speculation and what-ifs. It saved me a lot of aggravation.

I've developed a philosophy for dealing with fears and uncertainties about the future: "Don't worry about things until you know you have something to worry about." And there's a corollary: "If there is something to worry about, you'll have all the time in the world to worry about it then. You don't have to start early." These mottos have served me, and many of my patients, very well over time.

WHAT'S THE ALTERNATIVE?

The answer is not to ignore everything and bury your head in the sand. That kind of denial can be irresponsible or even dangerous. However, there is a middle ground between complacency and worry: concern.

On a spectrum it looks like this:

Complacency ←——————— Concern ———————→ Worry

Here's how I distinguish worry from concern:

Worry	Concern
Emotional	Intellectual
Fearful, anxious	Caring, interest
Problem-oriented (reactive)	Solution-oriented (proactive)
Stressful, draining	Appropriate, constructive
Hurtful	Helpful

In one of my seminars a man put it this way: "Worry is what I choke on; concern is what I *chew* on."

Instead of avoiding your fears, *confront* them, but in a constructive and organized way.

I've been using an exercise called Creative Worrying. It can be done whenever you're fretting about a particular issue. For example, if you're worrying about something at bedtime, you might do this exercise before you crawl into bed. Sit down with a pen and paper and answer these questions:

1. What's the worst thing that can happen? What's my greatest fear? (There, now you've said it!)

2. How likely is it to happen? What's the probability that this will actually occur?

3. If it does happen, what would I do to handle it? What measures would I take to deal with the problem?

4. What can I do now to either prevent it from happening or to prepare for it?

Once you've answered these questions, you have a game plan to implement if the worst really does occur. File it away and go to bed. There's nothing more that you can do right now. Further worry will provide absolutely no gain.

To keep things in perspective, remember the words of the French philosopher Montaigne: "My life has been a series of catastrophes—most of which never happened." If you're a chronic worrier, review your track record. Most of the things you worried about probably didn't happen. Notice that, even when certain things did happen, you dealt with them somehow and came through it. That's a helpful reality check.

- Notice what you worry about and when you worry (while driving? at bedtime?).
- Identify an issue that's stressing you right now: financial worries, relationship troubles, a health problem, job- or school-related issues, or anything else.
- Take a blank sheet of paper and confront your worries—don't run away from them.
- Do the Creative Worrying exercise in writing.
- Develop a plan to implement the ideas you generate for question 4.

David Posen, M.D.

Then file your sheet (and your worries) away and get back to your life!

Closing "Open Circuits"
Getting Closure on Unfinished Business

I T TOOK ME SOME TIME to fully understand the concept of a computer screen "desktop." I had documents, files and folders, but had to figure out how they all fit together and then how to access them. (You can tell I was older than twenty-five when I learned this technology.) Slowly I learned how to manipulate material, move files, have several documents open at once, flip back and forth, and use split screens. Once I caught on, I had the same sense of "eureka" that Archimedes felt in his famous bathtub. It was awesome!

But then I learned something else. I can only have so many screens on the go before I start to misplace things and feel disorganized (or before, as my son pointed out, the computer freezes). I realized there was a limit on how many files I could have open before I started to feel, well, *stressed!*

Just as we can get overwhelmed by multiple open computer files or juggling too many tasks at once, we can also be plagued by unresolved issues. They take up space in our heads and weigh us down emotionally. Stress can come not only from current events that hold center stage, but also from unfinished business that lurks in the wings. When patients come to see me, they usually have several issues that are generating stress. Most are recent, but some are long-standing—such as an unresolved conflict with a close friend years ago or regrets about not staying in school.

> There are three ways to close open circuits: pursue them, park them or pitch them.

"Closing open circuits" is a useful phrase I heard years ago. The more open circuits we have in our lives, the more potential there is for distraction, confusion and stress. Dealing with open circuits brings a sense of closure. Every problem we clear up takes one more issue off the table.

There are three ways to close open circuits:

- **pursue them** (to resolution)

- **park them** (for now)

- **pitch them** (let them go for good)

One man had promised his son a special trip, but the timing was never right, and years rolled by. It continued to nag at him. Finally, he decided to take the bull by the horns and make good on his commitment. They took their trip and had a great time together. He also got a bonus: a feeling of completion, and the satisfaction of having finally honored his promise.

The concept of closing open circuits has proved helpful to many of my patients. One woman was unhappy with her house—especially the location (location, location). She'd been wanting to move for years, and experienced almost daily feelings of irritation. After living with one foot out the door for a long time (which was very cold on winter nights, I suspect), she decided to stay put: "I've come to terms with my decision not to move. It's a nice house; it's fine—*for now*." She then put the issue out of her mind and got closure.

> Letting go of old baggage gives us freedom to truly live in the present moment.

Another man was struggling with relationship problems in his family that related to events that had happened decades earlier. He wanted to discuss these issues and work through them with his family, but no one else wanted to. He finally realized that he couldn't explore the problems further without their participation. He decided to stop his pursuit and move on. He had to close that chapter, even though it was unresolved, to leave it behind him so that he could move forward with his life.

- Make a list of issues you consider "unfinished business" (projects, relationships, events or feelings from the past).
- Pick one issue you'd like to confront and get closure on.
- Decide how best to resolve it:
  - If it's an unfinished project, complete it, or plan when you will finish. Or decide that it's not practical or worth the effort, and erase it from your list of "someday I'll get to that" items.
  - If it's a relationship issue, speak to the person or write a letter—clear the air, apologize, explain, clarify, make restitution—and resolve it. Or decide you can't (or aren't inclined to) deal with it—and let it go mentally and emotionally.
  - If it relates to old hurts, regrets or resentments, talk to a trusted confidante or professional and work through the issues. Or decide that you're ready to let the feelings go without resolution.

David Posen, M.D.

Tidying up loose ends is very satisfying. But choosing to let go of unfinished business, once and for all, can be equally beneficial.

The Art of Reframing

It's All in How You Look at Things

I WAS PRESENTING A MORNING WORKSHOP at a conference, one of several concurrent sessions before a gala luncheon. There were about a hundred people in my group, and things seemed to be going well for the first twenty minutes. Then a woman at the back of the room gathered up her purse and writing materials and quietly walked out. My immediate thought was, "Gee, I must have been a big hit with her." The moment passed, and I regained my confidence and carried on. An hour later the same woman reappeared, sat at the back of the room, opened her workbook and got involved in the session. After fifteen minutes she again picked up her things and left. This time I thought: "Strike two! She gave me a second chance, and I blew it." Again, I was taken aback, but quickly put it out of my mind.

At lunch all the speakers were seated at one table. And guess who was sitting with us? She came over to me and said, "Your session was terrific. I'm sorry I couldn't stay." ("Yeah, right!" I thought.) She continued, "I'm one of the (conference) organizers, and it was my job to slip in and out of the sessions to make sure things were under control. I could see your participants were really enjoying themselves. I wish I could have heard more." I was pleasantly surprised and relieved.

> We had to cancel a family vacation when our son got sick. My wife asked, "How can we reframe this?" I said, "Well, for one thing, we just saved $2,000!"

That incident became a touchstone for me, a reminder not to jump to conclusions. It also illustrates that most of our stress comes not from events and situations, but from how we interpret them. Things aren't always what they seem.

This raises an exciting possibility. If stress usually results from the way we think about things, then we can reduce our stress by *changing* the way we think. The technique for doing this is called **reframing**. It's one of the most powerful skills in our stress management repertoire.

139

We all reframe things at times, spontaneously and by instinct. Here's an example. In the 1970s, a postal strike in Canada went on for several weeks. Businesses couldn't send invoices, people couldn't send birthday cards and, where I worked in Oakville, Ontario, doctors couldn't mail letters to one another. Then someone had a brain wave: "Hey, we've all been looking at this as a problem. Why don't we turn it around? I think there's an opportunity here. We all have mailboxes at the hospital for our lab reports. Why don't we just bring our letters to the hospital and pop them in each other's mailboxes until the strike is over?" That creative solution worked very well. But guess what happened after the strike? Nobody went back to using the mail. To this day, Oakville doctors exchange letters at the hospital—same-day service, and it's free. The strike forced us to find a temporary solution, which turned out to be better than the system we were using. We weathered a crisis and found an unexpected benefit. This is a classic example of "necessity is the mother of invention." But it's also a form of reframing.

> If stress usually results from the way we think about things, then we can reduce our stress by changing the way we think.

We all reframe things on occasion, but we can learn to do it more consistently and by intention. When I was writing my first book, *Always Change a Losing Game*, it took me four years to find a publisher. When the first rejection letters came in, I got a little discouraged. So I developed other ways of looking at the situation:

- Reality check: "It's pretty unlikely that an unknown author would find a publisher on the first try. Obviously, the process takes time."

- "The longer I wait for an acceptance, the more exciting it'll be when it finally happens." This later proved to be true.

- "It'll make a much better story than if I'd found a publisher immediately." ("The Saga of How I Overcame Adversity.") Success is more interesting when it involves a struggle.

- "This is a test of my determination and persistence" (plus patience and optimism).

- "This gives me a chance to keep reworking my manuscript to make it better." As business guru and author Tom Peters observed: "Feedback is the breakfast of champions." In retrospect, I'm grateful the manuscript wasn't accepted in its early drafts. I think it's a much better book because of the time-consuming process that was required.

Reframing helped me to manage my frustration and disappointment. By seeing the rejections in a different light, those letters started to look like rungs on a ladder rather than rebukes from the universe. By changing my thoughts, I changed my feelings.

- Identify a situation that's upsetting you right now (the economy, a jerky boss or thoughtless neighbor, a project that's not going well).
- Ask yourself, "How else can I look at this situation? Is there another point of view I can take? What can this teach me?" Look for any positives, benefits or opportunities you hadn't seen before.
- Think of what you'd tell a friend in a similar situation (for example, "Why don't you think of it this way?").
- Ask a friend how she'd reframe it—or ask her to help you brainstorm other interpretations.
- Be playful. Ask, "Is there anything funny about this situation?"

David Posen, M.D.

Incidentally, if I'd discovered that the woman left my seminar because she thought I was doing a lousy job, I could have reframed that too—perhaps by saying, "Well, you can't please everybody all the time!"

Conversations with Yourself

Be Careful What You Say

ONE OF MY HIGHLY STRESSED patients was lamenting the pressures of his overloaded schedule. Among his many activities was volunteer work in a community organization. His position on the board required far more work than he'd expected. To lighten his load, I suggested he consider resigning his position. He said, "I can't do that. I'd feel like a quitter. I've never quit anything in my life."

His father had taught him to never give up or surrender in the face of a challenge—especially in sports or schoolwork. I suggested that he not get hung up on the word "quit." "Think of it as a necessary choice to take more control of your life and reduce your stress. I'm not saying you should 'quit'—only that you should 'resign.'" (Actually, the dictionary defines "quit" with words such as "to set free, depart from, leave, let go, discontinue," and "to stop doing a thing." All these words describe an action without making any character judgments. But "quit" *has* come to have negative connotations in today's society.) After our discussion, he gave notice that he would be leaving his volunteer position, a decision that now felt comfortable.

This story illustrates the connection between language and feelings. I once heard that "we use language, but language also uses us." Certain words are stress triggers or hot buttons, whereas other words evoke far less reaction. Making language distinctions can help to reduce stress.

I learned about using language from my mentor at Harvard, Dr. Matthew Budd. He wrote an excellent book on this subject called *You Are What You Say: A Harvard Doctor's Six-Step Proven Program for Transforming Stress Through the Power of Language* (movie fans take note: the introduction is written by Patch Adams, M.D.). It's a terrific book, combining great ideas and up-to-date brain research with a conversational style and a host of good stories. I highly recommend it!

We use language, but language also uses us.

Here are some distinctions in language that my patients have found helpful.

1. Assertive versus aggressive

Many people have difficulty speaking up for themselves and expressing their feelings. They fear they'll be seen as aggressive. So they choose to say nothing and become passive. Fortunately, there's a middle ground between these extremes: being assertive. Aggressive speech is forceful, loud, blunt or even attacking. Assertiveness is when you speak up for yourself without putting the other person on the defensive. It involves telling him how you feel by using "I" statements. So instead of saying, "You're rude and inconsiderate," you'd say, "I get frustrated when you don't return my phone calls." Or "I get upset when you're late for our appointments."

Different words generate different mindsets. "Being aggressive" feels uncomfortable for most people, whereas "being assertive" feels okay.

2. Feedback versus criticism

If something bothers me in a restaurant, I start with the phrase, "I'd like to give you some feedback. This is *not* criticism." Then I convey my message. I feel more comfortable—respectful, even virtuous. And the management is more receptive, usually thanking me because they hear it as helpful input. If giving negative information is difficult for you, stop thinking of it as criticism (which feels threatening) and present it as feedback (which is constructive).

3. Declining versus refusing

If you have trouble saying No, it may be the language you're using with yourself. Instead of thinking that you're "adamantly refusing" (which feels obstinate), think of yourself as "graciously declining." The fact is that you can't do everything that's asked of you or you'd quickly become overwhelmed. We all have to draw a line somewhere.

4. Relaxation versus laziness

A patient was blaming himself for his "laziness." Now a senior citizen, he felt the need to lie down and rest an hour after breakfast and again in the afternoon. He'd always been active and busy, so he was unhappy with his current behavior.

I felt he was being unfairly hard on himself. After all, he was in his seventies and retired. And he also had three serious diseases that left him tired and in constant pain. I was actually impressed by how well he was functioning and was captivated by his warmth and good humor. Laziness connotes sloth, indolence, and aversion to work—none of which applied to him. I said: "You're just lying down to relax and take it easy. That's not laziness." He found this distinction helpful, and started giving himself permission to do it without guilt.

> "The greatest discovery in our generation is that human beings, by changing the inner attitudes of their minds, can change the outer aspects of their lives."
>
> William James

This is an extreme case. But many other patients (especially the driven Type-As, who cut themselves no slack at all) have found this distinction useful as well.

℞
- Start to listen to the words you use this week. Notice their effect on you and on others.
- Pick a situation in which you'd like to give someone feedback, but feel uncomfortable (telling someone her answering machine message is too long, for example). Ask their permission: "Can I share a thought with you?" Then make a distinction: "This is feedback, not criticism."
- If someone makes a request you choose not to accept, think of yourself as "declining" rather than "refusing." It'll feel easier.
- Take a short time-out today and tell yourself how helpful it is to relax for a few minutes. Think of it as a well-earned rest, or a necessity to recharge your batteries. Banish the word "laziness" from your lexicon.

David Posen, M.D.

The words we use affect the way we feel. Talk to yourself differently and you'll reduce your stress. You'll also feel more freedom to act.

Thought Stopping
How to Stop Unwanted Thoughts

PICTURES OF WORK, PILED HIGH on your desk, dance through your mind at night. You've just had an argument with someone and can't get it out of your head. You have money worries, a sick child, a nagging boss or mice in the basement, and you can't stop thinking about it. Perhaps you're mulling over a problem, or ruminating about a past event. You analyze it in minute detail, worry incessantly or even wallow in self-pity. How do you get rid of this infernal racket in your head? There is a technique for stopping stressful thoughts that is deceptively simple—and it really works.

Don't you love it when someone goes on and on about something? Eventually you get irritated and think, "I wish he'd stop already!" In a way, this is what happens when your inner voice talks too much. The technique for dealing with this stressful monologue (in which you are both the talker and the listener) is called thought stopping. Just as you might say to a friend, "Can we talk about something else?" or even "Knock it off," you use a similar approach with yourself. But with a little more kick to it.

Here's how it works. First, notice when your mind slips into unwanted or stressful thoughts. Then yell something sharp and loud and jarring at yourself to interrupt the stressful conversation. Try words like, "Stop it!"; "Enough!"; "Cut it out!"; "Chill!" Use a forceful voice that will really grab your attention. Obviously, it's a good idea to do this when you're alone—in your car, in the shower, or when you're home by yourself. Try it for a few days to get the full impact. Then gradually quiet the messages until they're silent. I use the phrase, "That's enough, David!" (sub-vocally) when I catch myself with unpleasant thoughts. Another phrase in vogue these days is "Don't go there!" Anything will work, as long as it stops you in your tracks.

> If you use the technique of thought stopping and then sit there in a vacuum, the unwanted thoughts will likely return.

A colleague taught me a variation on this method. Place an elastic band around your wrist. When you start to experience upsetting thoughts, snap the elastic gently (for impact) as you say, "Stop it!" or "Enough." Three tips here: make sure the elastic band isn't too tight (you're not looking for a tourniquet here); snap it on the *back* of your wrist, not the sensitive underside; and don't pull the thing back like a slingshot—a small gentle snap is all that's needed.

Thought-stopping, however, is only half the story. If you use the technique and then sit there in a vacuum, the unwanted thoughts will likely return. So the second part of the exercise is to divert yourself. This can be a form of "thought substitution," where you purposely start thinking about something else—pleasant activities for the weekend, whom to invite for lunch or gift ideas for an upcoming birthday. Or you might think about your next vacation or the trip you took last summer.

"If you want to take your mind off your problems, try wearing tight shoes."

Thought stopping and thought substitution are especially useful if you awaken at night musing about work and have trouble shutting off the voice. If you can't get back to sleep, just lie quietly and think relaxing or pleasant thoughts. In one of my favorite images, I'm lying on the beach of a tropical island. I can see very clearly the white sand, the turquoise water, the bright sunshine and the palm trees waving gently in the breeze. It's a restful picture that helps me drift back to sleep.

To keep unwanted thoughts from recurring during the day, it helps to use some form of physical diversion. Pick up the phone and call a friend, grab a magazine or read your mail, turn on the radio or TV, look out the window, do a crossword puzzle or focus your mind on something stimulating or distracting.

The amazing thing about thought stopping and thought substitution is that, simple as they are, they're very effective. Patients have left me voice-mail messages over the years in which they've added at the end, "And, by the way, tell David that thought stopping really works!" It illustrates the extent to which we can take control of our thinking. We can't stop thoughts from popping into our heads. But we can choose how long we want to dwell on them.

• Start watching for worrisome or unpleasant thoughts that pop into your mind and trigger feelings of stress. Notice how long you hang on to these thoughts.
• Practice the thought-stopping technique, aloud, using whatever words you choose.
• Then shift your attention to other thoughts that are engaging and diverting.
• Repeat the process if the stressful thoughts re-emerge.
• Gradually soften the volume of your attention-getting word or phrase until it is silent.

David Posen, M.D.

The next time you want to tell someone to "Put a sock in it," you might be surprised to realize the person upsetting you is you! And you can actually silence that voice.

Reframing Other People's Behavior
It's Not Always About You

Y FORMER JUNIOR-HIGH PRINCIPAL told me a story about a boy sent to the office because he had thrown a snowball through a window (which, unfortunately for the kid, was closed at the time). The student knew he was in trouble, not only for the damage, but also for breaking a school rule. The principal sat him down and began by asking, "So tell me Bobby, what was going through your mind when you threw that snowball?" Totally disarmed (he'd expected to hear the riot act), the boy explained himself, while the principal listened with patience and respect. Then the principal said, "Thanks for helping me understand what happened. Is there anything else? Is everything okay at home?" And again, Bobby filled in some relevant background information. The principal then said, "It's helpful for me to know what contributed to this incident. Now, as you know, a school is a form of community, and communities have rules. And when rules are broken, there have to be consequences. What do you think would be a fair consequence in this situation?" He found that students would often come up with harsher punishments than anything he had in mind.

The result of this talk was that Bobby felt listened to, heard, understood and fairly treated. And, by handling discipline problems in this way, the principal learned more about what made his students behave as they did. What a much more enlightened way of dealing with children than simply bringing them into a room and bawling them out!

> We usually react not to what somebody does, but to our interpretation of why they did it.

There's an important lesson here about how we can reduce the stress of interacting with other people. We usually react not to what somebody does, but to our interpretation of why they did it. For example, you walk into work on Monday morning and say "Hi" to Joe—but he doesn't return your greeting. You feel a little hurt or insulted. Your feeling results not from Joe's lack of response, but from what you think it means. You may say to yourself, "I guess he's angry at me," or "He doesn't like me," or "He thinks I'm not very important." You're assuming his lack of reply reflects a negative feeling about you. Much of our interaction with others is based on this kind of judgment and self-talk.

> People's behavior is mostly about them, not about you.

It would be helpful at that moment to consider other possible reasons for Joe's behavior. Maybe he didn't hear you. Perhaps he was preoccupied with other thoughts, or personal problems that were weighing on his mind. Or perhaps he was just in a hurry. Given that your interpretation of his behavior is based on mind reading, guesswork and conjecture, you can't know with any certainty why Joe didn't acknowledge your greeting.

In discussions with patients, I often challenge their interpretations and ask them to think of other possible explanations for someone's behavior. One man went for a job interview. The meeting went well, and the interviewer told him he'd hear back by the end of the week. He didn't hear anything for ten days. His mind was filled with negative messages: he didn't have the job; the interviewer didn't care about his feelings; the company was unreliable. I asked him what other factors might explain why he hadn't been called. He came up with several possibilities: perhaps the selection process hadn't been as clear-cut as they expected; maybe new applicants had surfaced; a corporate emergency might have come up; the decision maker might be sick. Early the following week, he got a call to come in for another interview. The interviewer apologized for the delay—a family crisis had taken him away from work for several days. The applicant felt relieved. But during the stressful waiting period, it had helped him to reframe the situation, instead of assuming the worst.

We often jump to conclusions about why things happen—or *don't* happen—and get ourselves unnecessarily upset. The fact is that people's behavior is mostly about them, not about you. This is an important perspective to keep in mind. It will not only reduce your stress, but also help you to be a more open-minded, understanding person.

> "One of the nice things about being famous is that when you are boring, people think it's their fault."
> Henry Kissinger

- Think of a few situations in which you learned that you'd misread someone's motives or intentions.
- This week, start to observe how you talk to yourself about other people's behavior. Tune into your inner voice. Notice if you're frequently critical, or if you perceive someone's behavior as a snub or a dig.
- The next time someone offends or neglects you, think of reasons for their actions (or inaction) that have nothing to do with you. Ask yourself what might be going on in their life that would explain their behavior.
- Start to ask them questions. Then listen to their perception of reality, which will be different from yours. Listen to learn, not to judge.
- Notice whether your feelings toward them change. Monitor whether you feel less stressed around them.

David Posen, M.D.

My junior-high principal, Len Chellew, became a legend in Ontario education, admired by his colleagues and respected by his students.

Dealing with Difficult People
Stop Wishing They'd Go Away—They're Here to Stay!

ARLY IN MY TRAINING, I met a doctor who triggered a lot of stress in me. I found him arrogant, smug and full of himself. He also had a condescending, patronizing manner that I found offensive. It was bad enough when I ran into him only on occasion. But the capper came when I was assigned to work with him for two months. I couldn't imagine how I'd get through the ordeal.

As we started to work together, I found him less abrasive than I'd expected. Then something amazing happened. He asked me to work with him on a long case, and I found myself feeling flattered by the request. During our several hours together, I found myself lightening up and kibitzing a bit. He responded. By the end of the afternoon, we had made a breakthrough. That was a turning point, but it got even better.

As I got to know him, I enjoyed him more and more. Most important, I realized that he wasn't arrogant or smug at all. In fact, he was extremely shy and soft-spoken. What I had taken to be arrogance was the way he compensated for his social unease. His behavior and mannerisms didn't change, but my view of them changed completely. He became one of my favorite people, and we became real friends. This was a lesson in how easy it is for us to misinterpret other people, to react not to who they are, but to our interpretations and judgments of them.

> Even if you don't end up liking a person, getting to know him or her can lessen feelings of tension.

Here are some strategies that will help you deal with difficult people:

Appraisal

Learn where they're coming from and what makes them tick. The experience with the other doctor taught me that the more you know about someone, the better you understand her. Often her behavior becomes less irritating and upsetting.

Even if you don't end up liking her, getting to know her can lessen feelings of tension.

Avoidance

An obvious way to deal with stressful people is to just stay away from them. And where this is feasible, it usually works. However, it's not always possible to avoid people, particularly if you work or live with them. You may find yourself looking over your shoulder to make sure they're not nearby. This can be stressful in itself. Moreover, you can't learn how to deal with the person if you simply skirt the problem. Avoidance won't help you to develop better coping strategies. You could actually end up magnifying your stress when you *do* see her.

I learned this lesson years ago when I ran into someone I'd been studiously and stubbornly ignoring. He was sullen, abrasive and generally disliked, and I wanted nothing to do with him. One day I found myself walking toward this person with not another soul around. It would have been too obvious if I'd turned around and gone the other way. So I kept walking, determined not to make eye contact with him. I was going to show *him* what a jerk I thought he was! Well, guess whose stress level went up with every step? As I passed him, I noted with dismay (and, frankly, some amusement) what a lousy strategy I'd concocted. I felt *more* stress when I *couldn't* avoid him. After that, I realized avoidance wasn't the answer with this guy.

Appeasement

Give the other person what she wants in order to avoid conflict. This is the "line of least resistance" often employed by "pleasers." One of my patients used this approach with an aggressive friend of hers, saying that "being a pleaser is easier." However, she started to realize that appeasement wasn't really easier at all. It perpetuated her stress and gave her friend tacit permission to continue to be controlling, domineering and bossy. Appeasement may be necessary at times (to avoid a scene, for example), but isn't a great strategy on an ongoing basis. It keeps you feeling powerless and victimized.

> "Behave unto others as if they were about to become incredibly famous."
> Jay McInerney

Acceptance

Accept her as she is. You don't have to like her. Just acknowledge her characteristics in a neutral way, rather than judging and reacting.

Accommodation

Spend some time with her to find common interests and outlooks and build rapport. It may seem like a stretch, but you might be surprised at what emerges.

- Identify the difficult people in your life, and the traits that bother you.
- List the strategies you've tried for dealing with them up until now. How have they worked out?
- Consider other options. Learn more about them. Speak to people who know them, and try to understand what makes them tick.
- Spend some time just watching their behavior. Be an objective observer.
- Try to engage them in conversation about things that interest them and see if they warm up.

David Posen, M.D.

We've all had an experience in which someone we initially disliked turned into a good friend. I even know of cases where two people who disliked each other at their first meeting ended up getting married!

Stop Giving Power to Other People
There Are Gentle Ways to Push Back

ONE OF MY PATIENTS was having problems with her husband. While he could be charming at times, and was never physically abusive, he had a way of attacking her verbally on occasion, often unexpectedly. He would go into a tirade of berating and criticizing, making her feel small and unworthy. These attacks took a toll on both her self-esteem and her affection for him. I sensed that he wasn't a malicious guy and probably didn't realize how much harm he was doing her and their relationship.

One day I made a suggestion: "The next time he does that, why don't you listen as quietly as possible and, when he's finished, say to him, 'Thanks for sharing that with me,' and walk away." She burst out laughing and couldn't wait to try it. At her next visit, she reported what happened when she did. Her husband got all wound up and went into his spiel. She listened without getting upset. Then she delivered her quiet message in a dignified way, without sarcasm. He became flustered, embarrassed and totally deflated. For the next few weeks, he was a pussy-cat—pleasant, subdued and respectful.

> In taking control back from other people, aim for autonomy and self-determination, not power over them.

Then he reverted to form and started winding up to take another strip off her. This time, she preempted him. Feeling empowered from her success in the earlier confrontation, she said something totally out of character: "If you're going to have a temper tantrum, I'm going to sit here and watch. I can't get into this." And with that, she pulled over a chair, sat down and ceremoniously got herself comfortable. Then she looked up and said, "Okay, I'm ready." He stood there nonplussed, mumbled something and walked away. And, again, he became more pleasant toward her.

This woman finally realized that she didn't have to put up with his behavior. She'd been tacitly giving him permission to abuse her by not objecting. She had now found ways to break the cycle. Better yet, she could do so without provoking a fight.

Abusive behavior is a strategy used by some to control situations or other people. When I encourage patients to stop putting up with abuse, to take back the power they've given to others, I'm not suggesting that they take control (a role reversal that most people would be afraid to try), but that they stop participating in the perpetrator-victim struggle. I often use a Popsicle metaphor to make this point. In an uneven, power-wielding relationship, it's as if the abusive person has the entire Popsicle. The message you want to get across is not "I want the whole Popsicle," but "I don't want your half. I just want my half." In other words, "Let's share the Popsicle." The result is a more balanced relationship.

There are two kinds of control: over others (which I call "power") and over yourself (which I call "autonomy"):

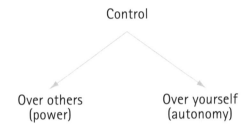

Control

Over others
(power)

Over yourself
(autonomy)

In taking control back from other people, aim for autonomy and self-determination, not power over them.

Abusive people are not as tough as we think. They seem confident and imposing, so we assume they have high self-esteem. Usually it's the opposite. In my experience, most abusive people feel insecure. They try to build themselves up by putting other people down. Whatever bluster or powerful facade they may project, they usually feel pretty small, or even frightened, on the inside, just like the Wizard of Oz—a small man with a powerful microphone hiding behind a curtain.

> "You don't fight to win but to clear the air and find a solution; to gain greater understanding and share feelings." Unknown

It's not just abusive people to whom we give power. We also give away control to folks with strong or dominant personalities. We let them take over meetings, monopolize conversations or make all our decisions. Before you give power to intimidating people, keep in mind that they're not as big and tough as you've made them out to be. And as soon as your backbone gets stronger, you'll see how quickly they retreat from their attempts to push you around.

An important way to deal with all these difficult people is to be assertive—speak up for yourself without attacking them. An assertive statement should

- use the pronoun "I" ("I find it hurtful when you say those things"; "I get upset when you raise your voice"; or even "I don't give you permission to treat me this way")

- tell them what you want ("I'd appreciate it if you'd word it this way" or "Please talk more quietly")

- tell them how they will benefit ("We'll be able to work better together" or "I'll have a clearer understanding of what you need from me")

Occasionally abusers will up the ante and escalate the abuse. But most often they back down when their victims stand up to them.

> **R̶x** • Identify a difficult or abusive person in your life (his abuse might be overt or subtle).
> • Identify the way(s) in which he's abusive (criticizing, insulting, yelling, embarrassing you in front of others, and so forth). Is there a pattern?
> • Plan what you will say to get him to change his behavior. Make some notes.
> • Decide on the best time to speak to him—when he next offends you or, pro-actively, before he repeats his behavior. Practice your assertive statements.
> • If the pattern of abuse persists or escalates, seek intervention by a third party or a professional.
>
> David Posen, M.D.

Clearing the air can have an amazingly beneficial effect on a relationship, and especially on your self-esteem. The woman who stood up to her husband never stood so tall!

Good Health—It's Your Choice

Be More Mindful of Your Choices

L ET ME BEGIN WITH A PREMISE: most of our behavior and activities are strategies designed to reduce stress. Before you think I don't get out much, or that I see everything through "stress-colored" glasses, let me explain.

What happens when we experience stress or feel upset? Some folks grab their favorite comfort food or light up a cigarette. Some people tell me the first thing they do when they get home at night is pour themselves a good, stiff drink to help them unwind from the day. Others withdraw and isolate themselves. Still others "dump their bucket" on arriving home, ventilating at length about the upsetting day they've just had. Some go out for a run, work in the garden or do yoga to release built-up tensions. Then there are those who veg out in front of the TV every evening. All of these (and this is only a partial list) are ways that people cope with stress. And while some are healthier or more constructive than others, all of them work to some extent or people wouldn't keep doing them.

But let's go further. Why do people leave early to get to appointments if not to avoid the stress of rushing and/or arriving late? Angry outbursts are a way that many people vent frustration. Crying and laughing are also tension relievers. For a lot of people, worrying is a subconscious strategy to deal with difficult situations. In fact, some individuals use worry as a conscious strategy to ward off trouble ("If I worry about it, it won't happen"). People often use procrastination to put off unpleasant activities or situations. Most of what we do can be looked upon as a coping strategy, conscious or unconscious.

> Most of what we do can be looked upon as a coping strategy, conscious or unconscious.

If this premise is true, then we should ask ourselves two questions:

1. Do our strategies work?

2. Are they causing any other problems?

Let's compare unhealthy coping strategies with healthy coping strategies:

Unhealthy	Healthy
Smoking	Exercising
Drinking alcohol	Relaxing
Overeating	Practicing good nutrition
Using drugs	Doing recreational activities
Withdrawing	Being assertive
Indulging in self-pity	Taking time-outs
Blaming	Using humor

Stress is one of the leading causes of ill health in our society. But, as if that's not bad enough, many of our coping strategies are, in themselves, unhealthy. So we're hit with a double whammy. We achieve two benefits by shifting from destructive coping strategies to constructive ones: 1) they're better stress reducers; and 2) they improve our health.

If we think of our bad habits not just as self-destructive lifestyle choices, but as misguided attempts to relieve stress, then we can start to look for better strategies that are both effective stress relievers *and* healthier for us overall.

Healthy lifestyle choices may not seem very sexy or exciting—but they sure have a big payoff!

So the next time you have a glass of wine to help you relax in a social situation or compulsively chomp on potato chips to reduce anxiety, stop and consider that you're actually trying to deal with stress. Then think of alternative ways to alleviate your stress, without the negative side effects.

• For the next week, observe your behavior and keep asking, "Why am I doing this?" Notice that many of your habits are intended to reduce stress in one way or another.

• Make a list of your coping strategies. Next to each item, note if it's healthy or unhealthy.

• Make a second list of just the positive or healthy choices. Then ask yourself what other constructive stress-reducing strategies you can try. Get ideas from your friends to add to your "Healthy Choices" list.

• Plan how and when (under what circumstances) you can best use these strategies.

• The next time you get upset, consult your list and consciously choose a healthier activity to reduce your stress.

David Posen, M.D.

I've been watching people (including myself) make lifestyle choices for over thirty years. When I started seeing those choices as (mostly subconscious) strategies to reduce stress, it gave me a whole new outlook on the way we live our lives. And again, I'm reminded that we have more control than we think. We just need to use that control more mindfully.

How I Learned to Meditate
A Personal Odyssey

A CONFESSION: WHEN I STARTED to do stress management counseling in 1981, I thought that relaxation techniques were flaky. I'd heard they were effective, but they seemed out on the fringe to me. I couldn't relate to them. Here's the story of my personal odyssey from skeptic to enthusiast.

When I decided, in 1985, to make stress management my full-time pursuit, I realized I needed to know more about relaxation skills. I enrolled in a course taught by Eli Bay, whom I'd met at a conference. My wife was interested as well, so we went together.

There were twenty people in the class. I fully participated in the sessions and did the homework assignments faithfully. But I felt detached from the group—and frankly a bit smug. My inner voice said, "I'm here out of academic interest, not because I really *need* this stuff!" However, by the third session I noticed something interesting: I was no longer clenching my jaw or grinding my teeth. Then it hit me: "Wake up, wise guy, there's something of value here for you too." With that shift in attitude, I became fully committed to the process. I completed the course with a considerable repertoire of relaxation techniques, many of which I still use to this day.

Fast-forward to 1996. By then I was a firm adherent to the principles of relaxation, and had referred many patients to the course. One day, a young man I was counseling told me he'd enrolled in a course on transcendental meditation. A few weeks later, he was meditating for twenty minutes twice a day. I asked how he found the time to do that. He replied, "When you get this much benefit out of something, you *make* the time." That really caught my attention. I decided to check it out myself.

"When you get this much benefit out of something, you make the time."

My wife joined me for the introductory lecture. They showed a video that featured the Maharishi Mahesh Yogi himself, as well as clips of several high-powered CEOs and celebrities who practiced meditation. One of them was football legend Joe Namath, who used to meditate in a corner of the dressing room before games. I thought, "Gee, if it's good enough for Broadway Joe the Jock, I'm in!" We signed up for the course. It finished on a Tuesday, and the next day we flew to the Bahamas for a vacation.

We arrived in Nassau at night, checked into our hotel and went to bed. The next morning I looked outside at the fabulous scenery and prepared to go to breakfast. My wife, Susan, pointed out that we had to meditate first. (The course advocates meditating for twenty minutes on waking in the morning and again in the afternoon.) I said, "Let's start when we get home. It's a beautiful day out there." Fortunately, she persisted. We delayed our breakfast and meditated.

That afternoon we were out on the beach, swimming, reading and enjoying the sun. Around 4:00, Susan said, "We need to go in and meditate again." There was no way I was going to go inside on such a gorgeous afternoon so, again, I resisted. We compromised: we decided to meditate on the beach. Now this was one busy place—scores of people, music, chatter, local folks selling everything from T-shirts to parasailing rides to hair-braiding. There, in the midst of all this chaos, we settled into our chairs and meditated. And, aside from all the external commotion, it was a pretty idyllic setting.

> I've gone from being a skeptic to an adherent to an advocate of relaxation and meditation.

We continued to do this for the rest of the week and after we returned home. Within a few weeks, I began to notice the benefits. I felt more calm and relaxed, and the activity itself was effortless and pleasant. It was a great way to start the day, and provided a wonderful break in the afternoon. I was hooked, and I still meditate regularly. I meditate quietly at home and at my office, but also on trains and planes, in the dentist's chair—just about anywhere.

An unexpected bonus was the number of times I've had creative thoughts while I'm meditating. It's a real discipline to keep from jumping up to write them down. However, I usually remember the ideas after I'm finished.

I've gone from being a skeptic to an adherent to an advocate of relaxation and meditation. They are life skills I wish I'd learned much earlier. But I'm sure I'll be practicing them for the rest of my life.

Relaxation Techniques

They're Pleasant and They Work!

T HE HUMAN BODY IS BEAUTIFULLY designed and balanced. Just as we have the ability to trigger a stress reaction when we feel threatened, we also have, hard-wired into our nervous system, an opposite physiological state of total relaxation. Harvard's Dr. Herbert Benson calls this "the relaxation response." It's not only a pleasant state to be in, but is an important natural antidote to the stress reaction, allowing our bodies to recover from and reverse the effects of sustained stress.

The relaxation response is the mirror opposite of the "fight-or-flight reaction." When we feel threatened, our heart rate speeds up, our blood pressure rises, our breathing gets faster, our muscles tense, and so on. When we're in a relaxed state, our heart rate slows down, our blood pressure falls, our breathing gets slower and deeper, and our muscles loosen up. However, unlike the stress reaction, which is involuntary and triggers automatically, the relaxation response has to be brought forth voluntarily and by intention. This means that we have to choose to become relaxed in order for it to happen. Fortunately, there are many ways to do this that are easy to learn: meditation, yoga, self-hypnosis, visualization and others.

In the relaxation response, unlike in sleep, the body is fully relaxed, but the mind is alert and under conscious control. The goal is to "quiet the mind," slowing down thoughts and concerns and simply *existing* in a relaxed state. To prevent distracting thoughts, you can concentrate on a mantra, or on your breathing or on calming, repetitive images.

"When you breathe as if you are relaxed, you become relaxed."
—Jill Bay

While relaxation techniques can be learned from books or tapes, I think the best way of acquiring these skills is to take a course. It gives you hands-on teaching and practice, along with structure and support if you have problems with self-discipline. I recommend that couples take the course together, to increase their commitment and to give support to each other.

In the meantime, here are some easy-to-learn exercises to get you started.

RELAXATION (DEEP OR ABDOMINAL) BREATHING

Relaxation breathing is probably the simplest relaxation exercise because it focuses on a natural body function. It can be performed on its own, or combined with other techniques. It gets its name from the fact that we breathe differently when we're stressed than when we're relaxed. Under stress, the chest expands, the shoulders rise, and we breathe rapidly in order to take in air quickly. This is sometimes called "military breathing" (as in "chest out, tummy in, look smart!"). During relaxation, the abdomen expands with each breath in. This is the way we all breathed when we were infants, and how we still breathe when we're asleep. And as Eli Bay of The Relaxation Response in Toronto observes, "When you breathe *as if* you are relaxed, you *become* relaxed."

"I've tried relaxing, but—I don't know—I feel more comfortable tense." Unknown

Here's how it's done:

- Breathe in through your nose and out through your nose or mouth (opened slightly).

- Breathe into your abdomen. Feel your tummy rise as you inhale and fall as you exhale.

- Breathe slowly—otherwise, you'll hyperventilate.

- Start by breathing out to empty your lungs in preparation for the first deep breath.

- Focus on and observe your breathing (this is a form of self-hypnosis).

- If you're having trouble, put one hand on your tummy and the other hand on your chest. As you breathe, focus on the abdominal hand moving and the upper hand staying still on your chest.

PROGRESSIVE (MUSCLE) RELAXATION

Progressive relaxation was first described by Edmund Jacobson, a Chicago physician. In his 1929 book, called *Progressive Relaxation*, he described a technique of deep muscle relaxation that reverses the muscle tension of a stress reaction. This way of accessing the relaxation response involves focusing on different muscle groups and consciously letting them relax.

It goes like this:

- Start from your toes and work up, going slowly and with conscious awareness.

- Focus your attention on the muscles of your toes and allow them to relax.

- Then move your attention to the muscles of your feet and let them relax.

- Move up to your ankles, then your shins, calves, knees, and so on, until you have focused on every muscle group in your body.

- As you let go of tension in each muscle group, continue to be aware of the muscles you've already relaxed, so that you can feel the wave of relaxation rising in your body.

- Find a quiet, comfortable environment. You can sit or lie down.
- Loosen tight clothing, remove your shoes and glasses, and get fully comfortable.
- Close your eyes.
- Practice relaxation breathing for five minutes to start, then slowly increase to fifteen or twenty minutes throughout the week.
- Once you feel comfortable with relaxation breathing, try progressive muscle relaxation on alternate days.
- For maximum benefit, practice regularly (preferably every day).
- You can also use the skills on an "as needed" basis (before a job interview or before giving a presentation), and for as little as three to five minutes.

David Posen, M.D.

Relaxation techniques are safe, portable and natural and have no negative side effects. They are easy to learn and pleasant to do, and there are multitudes of different techniques to choose from. And, best of all, they work!

Outlets for Frustration

Alternatives to "Jumping out of Your Skin"

I N MY LATE TEENS I WORKED at a summer camp 300 miles north of Toronto. I drove up with a fellow counselor and, after a long first day, we finally stopped at a motel for the night. It was 2:00 a.m. when we checked into our room. A minute later, I noticed my friend wandering across the parking lot toward the office.

"Where are you going?" I asked him.

"I'll be back in a minute, Dave."

"Where are you going?"

"To use the phone."

"Who you gonna call at this hour?"

(Hesitation) "My mother."

"What for?"

"To tell her where we are."

"You're gonna wake her up just to tell her that you're here?"

"She's not asleep."

"How do you know?"

"She won't go to sleep until she hears from me."

"You're kidding!"

"I'm telling you, Dave, she'll be up."

> We need channels to drain off our restlessness and agitation.

"Doing what?"

"Probably the laundry. When she's worried or upset she'll stay up half the night ironing or washing the floor."

Fast-forward about thirty years. When I was extremely upset I could spend hours fixing up the basement or an entire evening cleaning out the garage. I was doing what my friend's mother was doing: getting rid of excess stress energy. When we're under stress, our bodies are wound up like tightly coiled springs. It's hard to sit in one place, much less relax or go to sleep. My wife calls it "feeling like I'm going to jump out of my skin."

It's at times like this that we need channels to drain off our restlessness and agitation. Dr. Robert Sapolsky of Stanford University calls these "outlets for frustration." Most of us find something that is physically active and mentally distracting. When people start pacing around the room, shuffling paper or organizing their sock drawer, they're often just keeping busy to siphon off high levels of stress energy.

For nine years, I played trombone in our local orchestra. No matter how stressed I was from work, within a half hour of playing my horn, it would all melt away.

Here are some constructive outlets for frustration:

- **Physical activity:** Raking leaves, shoveling snow, working in the garden or cleaning out the basement, garage, kitchen cupboards or clothes closets will help. Punching a pillow or hitting a punching bag (no home should be without one) or hitting golf balls are other forms of physical release. If you pick tasks like chopping wood, you'll be doing something useful while you're dissipating your stress.

- **Exercise or sports:** A brisk walk, run or bike ride; squash; tennis; an aerobics class or gym workout—even dancing—can help you unwind.

- **Relaxation:** It can be difficult to sit and relax when you're feeling all wound up, but sometimes it works. Watching TV or flipping through a magazine might help you unwind. Relaxation breathing and meditation help to neutralize the stress reaction and calm you down.

- **Massage:** Although someone else does the work while you relax, massage is a terrific way to get rid of muscle tension (although it's not always available on short notice).

- **Ventilation:** Talking to another person is very helpful—find someone who's a good listener. Just getting things off your chest can be both calming and healing. Katharine Hepburn had another form of ventilation: I've heard that she used to drive her car out into the countryside, roll down the windows and just yell for a while to get it all out. Then she'd roll up the windows and drive calmly back to town.

- **Humor:** Laughter is a terrific way to relieve tension. Playing with kids or kibitzing with friends can be restorative. Funny magazines or books, cartoons, TV sitcoms and funny movies are great stress relievers.

- **Diversion and distraction:** Crossword puzzles, jigsaw puzzles, woodworking, sewing, knitting and other hobbies occupy your mind and your energies.

- Music: When I was in university, I spent endless hours playing the piano or guitar for stress relief (and as a way to goof off from studying). Listening to music is another outlet. Sometimes rock music works well; at other times, classical music produces a calming effect.

- **Prayer:** For many people, reading spiritual texts or practicing religious customs can be very beneficial.

> - Think of your own experiences. Which outlets for frustration have been most helpful? Which ones do you gravitate toward?
> - From your own list or the one above, pick one new outlet to try this week when you feel the tension building up.
> - Continue the intervention until you feel calm enough to resume your previous activity.
> - In the next few weeks, experiment with new and different ways to relieve stress. Expand your repertoire.
>
> David Posen, M.D.

It will be only the rare time that you'll stay up half the night to get rid of stress energy. But if that happens, you'll sure work through a pile of laundry!

Dealing with Anger
Getting Angry Is a Reaction; Staying Angry Is a Choice

S ATURDAY MORNING. A BUSY EXECUTIVE is waiting for important documents that are being sent by courier. They're supposed to arrive by noon. Shortly after 12:00, he finds out the package won't be delivered until Monday. He'd set aside this time to work on a project with a tight deadline. He is not pleased!

This tale is not about working on the weekend or unreliable couriers. It's about what happens next. The man (who admits to having high control needs) becomes angry. Very angry. Angry to the point of throwing things (although nothing breakable nor thrown at anyone). He stays angry for two hours.

This story illustrates three points:

- Anger is a normal emotion, common to us all.

- Anger involves behavior. How we express anger is a choice.

- How long we *hang onto* anger is also a choice.

Anger in itself is not the problem—although it can raise blood pressure dramatically in certain people known as "hot reactors." But how angry we become, how we manifest it and how long we stay angry can be very serious problems—for ourselves and for others.

> We can train ourselves to tolerate frustrations and irritations without getting angry.

Kids can teach us a lot about managing anger. They express their feelings openly and then let them go. They get frustrated or upset, but within minutes they're laughing and playing, leaving the anger behind. They're great at living in the moment.

There are many ways to deal with anger in acute situations. One is to ignore what happened or choose to shrug it off ("I'm not gonna let this get to me" or "This isn't worth getting upset about"). *You don't have to react* just because someone does something you don't like.

168

Another approach is to pause and reflect on the situation. Then you can tactfully respond without attacking the person who triggered your anger: "I'm really angry and I want to tell you why."

A third approach is to defuse the anger through diversion, distraction, humor or by talking about it (to yourself or someone else) in a way that helps you to understand why you're upset and to calm you down.

Dealing with anger can be thought of as a series of choices:

1. **Get angry or don't.** Anger is a reaction, but it's not inevitable. We can train ourselves to tolerate frustrations and irritations without getting angry—to accept things as they are and to accept that events don't always work out as we'd like and people don't always behave the way we think they should.

2. **Acknowledge or deny it.** Some people say "I'm not angry" when they really are, which can confuse both others and themselves. If you are angry, admit it—at least to yourself.

3. **Prolong it or let it go.** Anger (especially over small things) usually dissipates quickly. But hanging onto it (especially intentionally) prolongs your upset. It's self-indulgent, self-defeating and potentially self-destructive.

4. **Repress or express it.** Holding anger in too long is not healthy. It builds up internal pressure and ongoing stress. Expressing anger constructively (ventilation) is healthier.

5. **Express it directly or indirectly.** Direct ventilation is when you express your anger to the person involved—face to face, by phone or in writing. You can do it immediately or after some time. You can do it in a calm, assertive way or an angry, aggressive way. I suggest the former because aggressiveness can cause hurt feelings or escalate conflict. Direct expression of anger should be done carefully and, preferably, after you've calmed down.

Indirect expression of anger can be verbal, written or physical. It's safer because it avoids direct confrontation. Verbal ventilation can be done by talking to yourself, another person or even a pet. The objective is to unburden yourself—get the feelings out and let them go. Expressing your feelings can also help you to clarify why you're angry. (You might even realize that your anger is mostly at yourself.)

Expressing anger in writing can be very therapeutic, whether in a journal, a diary or an angry letter written to the person in question. If you're going to write an angry letter:

- Do it only when you're actually angry (to discharge the anger), not when you're feeling good (which only stirs up the anger).

- Say anything you damn well please: expletives, insults—anything to get it off your chest.

- Write quickly. Don't worry about legibility.

- *Don't send the letter.* The point is to express your thoughts, not to share them.

- *Don't reread the letter.* Roger Mellott, a stress therapist in Louisiana, uses the phrase "marble dumping" to describe ventilating anger. He likens getting angry to swallowing heavy marbles (think ball bearings) and having them sit in your stomach. When you ventilate anger, you're getting rid of those marbles. When you're finished, you feel lighter and relieved. However, if you reread the letter, you'll simply swallow the marbles all over again. The objective is to get the anger out, not to admire your handiwork afterward.

- *Destroy the letter.* Writing the letter was the exercise. It's already served its purpose. Now get rid of it for safety's sake.

Physical ventilation drains off the stress energy from anger. Exercise, sports or a physical activity like mopping floors or chopping wood (watch your toes if you're really angry!) can all do the trick.

"You will not be punished for your anger. You will be punished by your anger."

Anger serves a purpose. It helps us recognize when something's wrong (such as when we're being abused or exploited). But some people get angry over minimal situations or frustrations. This kind of anger is not helpful.

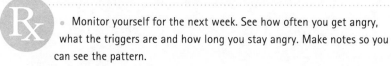

- Monitor yourself for the next week. See how often you get angry, what the triggers are and how long you stay angry. Make notes so you can see the pattern.
- Pick a situation that triggers anger for you (slow drivers, for example) and choose to let it go.
- The next time you get angry, step back, take a few breaths or count to ten and analyze why you're upset (feeling frustrated, wronged, a loss of control, embarrassed, etc.)
- Then think of a tactful, constructive way to handle the situation. Respond thoughtfully rather than react impulsively.
- See how quickly you can let go of your anger. Avoid angry silences or trying to punish others with your anger.
- **If you get angry frequently or are unable to control your anger, seek professional help.**

David Posen, M.D.

If you want a role model for letting go of anger, watch a little kid throw a temper tantrum and be laughing five minutes later. Then see if you can match that—preferably without the tantrum.

Dealing with the Blues
How to Get Up When You're Feeling Down

HAVE YOU EVER BEEN IN A FUNK and had someone try to "jolly" you out of your doldrums? They say something like "Come on, buck up. It can't be that bad" (and you say to yourself, "Wanna bet?"). Or it's "Snap out of it. Let me see you smile" (and your inner voice says, "Back off buddy. Don't press it!"). These people may mean well, but you'd still like to bop them, right? How about the ones who even go so far as to push up the sides of your mouth into a phony smile (and you think, "Watch your fingers!"). Don't you wish these folks would stop being so "helpful"?

These well-intentioned people are making at least two mistakes. First, they're intruding on your inner space without asking permission. Second, they're assuming that the simple injunction "Feel better" is enough to change your mood.

The fact is that it's difficult to change how you feel by a simple act of will.

California psychiatrist Dr. William Glasser taught a valuable concept during a seminar I attended years ago. He noted that we all function on four levels: doing, thinking, feeling and physiological response. And we have increasingly less control as we go down the list. Thus we have most control over our actions, less over our thoughts, very little over our feelings and even less over our physiological reactions.

> Even though you can't change your mood directly, you can change it indirectly—by changing what you do and the way you think.

Here's an illustration. You wake up on a Saturday morning feeling down. A friend calls to invite you to play tennis. You tell him you're not in the mood. He replies, "I'm sorry to hear that. But maybe playing tennis will give you a lift. I'll pick you up at 10:00." Despite your funk, you could put on your tennis gear and grab your racket. By mechanically putting one foot in front of the other, you could make yourself go out and play.

Or your friend could say, "I know you've been feeling down lately. But being inactive and staying alone is probably not going to help. I've read that physical activity and interaction with other people can actually help improve your mood. I think it's worth a try. It's a beautiful day and once you start beating me, you'll probably feel much better." By appealing to your rational self, he could help you to *think* differently about how to manage your mood. And even if you're unenthusiastic, you could accept his logic.

However, if this friend said to you, "Oh, come on, just feel better. Be happy," it would probably do nothing to improve your mood (although it could well add a level of irritation to your depression). You couldn't just push a button and suddenly feel fine.

In other words, you can change your actions and your thinking by volition, but you can't change your mood simply by deciding to change it.

Another important message from Dr. Glasser was that, even though you can't change your mood directly, you can change it indirectly—by changing what you do and the way you *think*. By doing and thinking differently, you can actually start to feel different. This is the premise behind behavioral and cognitive therapy. So if you go out to play tennis with a friend, or go for a walk on a sunny afternoon, it's very possible that you'll start to feel better (even in spite of yourself).

Changing the way you think is a proven and powerful way to lift your mood. When people feel depressed, they start to engage in negative self-talk. They think negatively about their situation and the larger world, about themselves and about the future. Talking this out with another person can help to put things into perspective. You can start to realize that things aren't as bad as you perceived and that there are positive aspects you've been ignoring.

"I've learned that if you want to cheer yourself up, you should try cheering someone else up."
Unknown

Rx
· The next time you're feeling down or depressed, identify and acknowledge the mood you're in.

· Ask yourself, "What is one thing I can do today to cheer myself up?" Pick at least one constructive activity (going for a walk, playing a musical instrument, working at a favorite hobby, meeting a friend for lunch, going to a movie) to divert your attention and help you feel better.

· Figure out what's bothering you. It may help to talk it through with another person or explore it in writing. See if you can identify why you're upset. Then try to uncover the thoughts behind the upset.

· Challenge those thoughts. Are they illogical, exaggerated, inaccurate?

· **If these measures are not successful, and especially if your depressed mood lasts more than two weeks, seek professional help from a family doctor or therapist.**

David Posen, M.D.

If you want to help people cheer up, invite them out for a walk or a bite of lunch. Just don't try to push their mouths up into a smile. There are teeth behind those lips!

The Importance of Social Support
A Problem Shared Is a Problem Halved

CHRIS MICHALAK WAS ONE of the real feel-good stories early in the 2001 baseball season. Michalak was a rookie pitcher with the Toronto Blue Jays. He began the year by beating the New York Yankees twice and winning his first three games. But what's most notable about Michalak is that he was thirty years old and had spent eight years in the minor leagues.

Many stories were written about Chris's determination, persistence and patience while trying to get his professional career on track. And in most of these articles and interviews, Michalak made a point of paying tribute to his wife, Sharon, whose support was invaluable to him, especially over the last four years of struggle. However difficult those years may have been, the fact that she believed in him and continued to encourage him was crucial to his success. This story illustrates the importance of support systems in our lives.

Here's another example. A friend of mine just had her first book published, a wonderful and satisfying accomplishment. It was also an occasion for celebration. Her husband and children pulled together a spectacular party with great entertainment and an even bigger surprise—two of her siblings flew over from Europe for the event. What made the affair so memorable and meaningful was that it was shared with dozens of loving relatives and friends— who were celebrating the author herself, not just her book.

People who suffer alone suffer a lot.

Social support is most helpful at times of stress. Many studies show that social support decreases the stress hormones in our bodies. My children have had several surgical procedures in their young lives, and even though I'm a doctor, these are times when I can do nothing for them medically. I have to leave that part to my surgical colleagues. But what I can do is to be there with them. The unspoken message is "I can't always protect you from pain, but I can stay with you when you have to experience pain so that you won't be alone." My wife and I see our role as giving comfort, providing distraction, giving reassurance, answering questions, allaying fear, and even, when appropriate, being kibitzers and trying to get the kids to laugh. Sharing difficult times together made those experiences more manageable and also brought us closer together as a family.

Self-help groups can be very beneficial for people with specific health problems, such as depression, obesity, heart disease or diabetes. Some studies have shown that women with breast cancer have better outcomes when they participate in support groups with other breast cancer patients. With alcoholics, the most effective treatment program has been Alcoholics Anonymous. Members provide acceptance, understanding and support at regular meetings. They also celebrate milestones of sobriety. The support is most meaningful because it comes from other alcoholics who know exactly how hard it is to overcome this addiction.

"Just keep giving and the taking will look after itself."

Harry Posen

In his excellent book *Love and Survival*, Dr. Dean Ornish notes that people who have close relationships and a strong sense of connection and community enjoy better health and live longer than those who live in isolation or alienation. My motto is that people who suffer alone suffer a lot.

The benefits of social support include:

- **Emotional support and encouragement:** A shoulder to lean on and an ear to listen are essential. Talking about feelings (ventilation) reduces stress and helps us work through problems and feel better about ourselves.

- **Logistical support:** At times of overload, illness or injury, other people can take care of our children, help with tasks or errands, or drive us to medical appointments.

- **Mentoring and coaching:** After a job loss or relationship breakup, people who have been through a similar experience can share the lessons they've learned. Others can also show us how to use a computer, build a deck, write a résumé or prepare for an interview.

- **Networking:** People in our support system can tell us about a job opportunity, a good car mechanic or a new book club.

A lot of people have difficulty opening up to others. Many patients tell me they feel weak or vulnerable when they admit to having problems. Or they don't trust people to keep the information confidential. And yet, as hairdressers, bartenders and taxi drivers will attest, people often reveal surprisingly personal information to total strangers.

Interestingly, many patients who don't share their feelings tell me that other people often confide in *them*—and that they feel flattered and enjoy being helpful. Yet they're reluctant to discuss their own personal lives or feelings.

The best *time* to develop a support system is before you need it. Don't wait till you're halfway up the twist and then run out to some passerby on the street and say, "I have to tell you about my day!" And the best way to develop a support system is to give support to others. This establishes a relationship and builds trust and goodwill. When you know someone is upset, ask if he'd like to talk about it. Then listen patiently and empathically. Call or visit someone who's sick or going through a rough time. Then, when you need a listening and caring ear, you'll have built a connection that can be reciprocated comfortably. As my father put it, "Just keep giving and the taking will look after itself."

> "Silent company is often more healing than words of advice."
> Unknown

- Identify people whom you trust and who care about you. Pick one person to talk to this week.
- Confide only what's comfortable for you. You don't have to divulge your entire life story. Venting feelings is more important than sharing details.
- Start to develop or expand your support system. Pick one person to reach out to and connect with, perhaps by offering your own support.
- Ask for help when you need it. Most people are happy to help.
- Turn to professionals for certain problems—a family doctor, a member of the clergy or a trained therapist.

David Posen, M.D.

Don't judge yourself as "less than" when you seek support. We all feel stressed, angry, frustrated or scared at times. It's a mistake to keep those feelings in. Having problems doesn't mean you're weak. It means you're only human.

How to Enjoy Holiday Stress

Be Proactive—Plan Ahead

C HARLES DICKENS BEGAN *A Tale of Two Cities* with the line, "It was the best of times, it was the worst of times." Paraphrased for the holiday season, it could read "I can't wait for Christmas—to be over!"

A radio survey a few years ago revealed that the number one stressor at Christmas time is "finding enough time to fit everything in." For many folks, especially women, Christmas is a four-letter word, and it's not spelled X-M-A-S. It's W-O-R-K! December is usually crammed with shopping, entertaining, visiting, decorating, sending cards, cooking, baking—and cleaning up.

I've observed Christmas through the eyes of my patients for over thirty years—and have watched the stress, exhaustion, mixed feelings and even anguish that can arise at this time of year. Surely there are better ways of handling the "festive season," whether you celebrate Christmas, Hanukkah, Kwanzaa or other holidays.

WHERE DOES HOLIDAY STRESS COME FROM? WHAT CAN WE DO TO MANAGE IT BETTER?

1. Gift buying

Holiday shopping in December—ahh, the memories: fighting for a parking space; elbowing your way through crowded stores; getting overheated from wearing your winter coat indoors (taking it off just means one more thing to carry); finding out they don't have the size or color you want; the person ahead of you taking the last piece of cut glass just as you reach for it; the sales staff nowhere in sight or too busy to help; forgetting where you parked your car. Are you having fun yet?

The perfect Christmas is an illusion.

The solution is to shop early—like in October! You do risk paying full price for stuff that will be marked down on December 23 and thinking, "If only I'd waited." But, of course, if you *had* waited, that would be the year they sold out in November. I buy gifts throughout the year—whenever a great idea grabs my attention—and stash them away.

Ask family members to prepare gift lists. Use catalogs to get ideas and to order gifts in advance. Consider shopping online. Do comparison shopping by phone. Stop trying to find the "ideal" gift. Give gift certificates to hard-to-buy-for people. Consider magazine subscriptions or gift coupons for a massage or movie. Give gifts of yourself (a booklet of your favorite recipes, for example).

2. Greeting cards

Sending out greeting cards can be a real "make-work" project. I've watched patients scrambling in mid-December to send out dozens of cards. Internal debates abound: Do I send a family picture? Shall I write a personal message in each card? Should I write a separate letter or send a newsletter? Or send an e-greeting card by e-mail? The key is to do what you can handle and what feels comfortable. If it's not pleasurable, why bother?

Decide how many cards you can realistically send. Prune your list from last year. Start by eliminating all the names you no longer recognize. Don't send cards to people you'll be seeing during the holidays. Don't get carried away with long letters. Start early. Do a few at a time. Pace yourself.

3. The social whirl

As if planning, shopping and preparing aren't enough, many people add a blitz of socializing to the holiday mix. The result is overload and exhaustion. Don't accept every invitation you receive. Give yourself some evenings off to relax and go to bed early. Don't accept two invitations for the same evening (the "we'll try to drop in" syndrome). Be realistic about travel time.

Keep regular hours and routines as much as possible. Get adequate sleep. Avoid excesses. Don't overeat, drink too much and then tank up on caffeine so you can drive home. When the little voice in your head says, "I think you've had enough," listen up, especially when it comes to alcohol consumption. Arrange for a designated driver. Stick to the "one drink per hour" rule. Have a nonalcoholic beverage (water is best) between alcoholic drinks.

4. Unrealistic expectations

The perfect Christmas is an illusion. And the quest for perfection is guaranteed to end in frustration and disillusionment, because nothing will measure up. Some people have mythical ideals about the holiday season or gilded memories of when everything seemed to be warm and wonderful. They try to recreate the feeling of remembered Christmases. These images are often more romanticized than real.

- Don't compare with past years. This is not a contest. Don't try to make every Christmas "the best ever." Just take it as it comes and enjoy it on its own terms.

- Don't strive for "the perfect Christmas." The house doesn't have to be spotless. Not every meal has to be prepared from scratch. It's really okay to go out and buy the dessert instead of cooking your own cake or pie. Remember two phrases: "When all else fails, lower your standards" and "Dare to be average."

Everyone has beliefs about the holiday season (you don't open gifts until Christmas morning, the tree has to be green, etc.). You don't have to create the kind of Christmas you had as a child. Start new traditions and create new memories. One of my former nurses developed a ritual of making gingerbread men to hang on the tree and to give to friends. Each of her children got a new pair of pajamas to open on Christmas Eve. Another family started a tradition of going to church on Christmas Eve and then coming home to watch a holiday movie.

It all comes down to starting early and managing your expectations.

It's also unrealistic to try to please everyone or do everything for everybody. This is especially a trap for women, who are socialized to meet the needs of others. Don't try to be all things to all people. Take that burden off your shoulders. Don't tie yourself into a Christmas wreath trying to be Superwoman.

5. Preparations, cleanups and chores

One of my patients decided to paint her front hallway the week before Christmas because she was having company. She must have read my mind because, without a word from me, she said, "Bad idea, huh?" She realized the timing for this make-work project was far from ideal.

One way to reduce the holiday workload is to *avoid all unnecessary tasks.* Keep it simple. You aren't entertaining royalty. If people ask if they can bring something, say yes! Sharing the load is both sensible and helpful. If they don't offer, consider asking for help or delegating some tasks. But be careful who you delegate to—and give clear instructions. A woman told me that her husband volunteered to buy the turkey. But when he proudly presented the bird, late on December 24, it was still frozen. No way would it defrost overnight. And, by then, all the stores were closed. He spent that Christmas with egg on his face.

Sharing the work includes the cleanups. We have friends who have a tradition for special dinners. When the meal is over, the two brothers disappear into the kitchen, roll up their sleeves and wash all the dishes before anyone realizes what's happened. These are the guests from heaven. (And, no, I won't give you their names. They're coming to *our* house this year!)

R℞
  • Sit down and think about how you want to "do" the holidays this year (exchanging gifts, entertaining, socializing, etc.).
  • Think about last year. What went well? What didn't? Pick one or two changes for this year so the festivities will be more pleasing to you—and easier to manage.
  • Make a schedule for gift shopping, sending cards and entertaining company.
  • Pace yourself. Allow yourself to enjoy the holiday season.

David Posen, M.D.

There is no one so calm (or smug) as the person who's done all her shopping, trimmed the tree, mailed her cards and planned her social calendar by early December.

By starting now, that person could be you!

Feelings That Surface During the Holiday Season

'Tis the Season to Be Jolly—or Just Emotional

A FRIEND TOLD ME about a Christmas morning fiasco at their house. They all went to bed early on Christmas Eve, with everything organized for the morning. At 7:00 a.m. they were jolted awake by a scream, followed by loud crying. Their five-year-old daughter had gone into the living room to discover a scene of utter chaos. Her three-year-old sister was so excited about opening presents that she couldn't sleep. At 5:00 a.m., unable to contain herself, she'd opened every gift (hers and everybody else's) and left everything strewn all over the floor. The parents hurriedly restored order by rewrapping all the packages and putting them back under the tree.

This story illustrates how the focus on gift giving can create a level of anticipation and excitement that can get totally out of hand. (I know some adults who get pretty pumped up too!) Expecting to receive certain gifts can lead to letdown if you don't get what you want. Or the giver can feel slighted if he gets the wrong reaction to his carefully selected treasures. A friend gave her grandfather a necktie that she thought was rather elegant. He was a really sweet guy and meant no offence, but he blurted out, "I wanted *cuff links*!"

A lot of emotions surface during the holiday season. There are happy feelings. There is solemn reverence for the religious aspect of the season. The beauty and pageantry often evoke feelings of warmth and connection. But other emotions surface that are difficult to manage: sadness, loneliness, feelings of loss, longing for the past, depression, family tension and conflict, anger or feelings of rejection. The holiday season can also be a divisive time as families decide which relatives to visit. I remember two patients having a tug of war in my office between the husband's family in Owen Sound and his wife's relatives in Kitchener. It almost seemed easier to stay home!

Then there are "the relatives." Aunt Martha, who keeps kissing everybody, Uncle Edgar, who tells every joke he's heard in the past year (including the off-color ones), and cousin Frankie, who drinks too much and embarrasses everyone.

For some people the feelings are those of pressure and apprehension. A patient of mine was troubled because she believed, "I am responsible for everyone having a happy Christmas." I saw her on December 23, and she was dreading Christmas Day. She had put tremendous pressure on herself to make sure everybody had a good time. We discussed how unrealistic this was and how unfair it was to her. I gave her permission to give up that self-appointed role for this particular Christmas. I said, "You've invited everyone over, you've done a ton of work, you're providing the food and a nice atmosphere. Let them be responsible for enjoying themselves." In January she told me that she took my advice and had the best Christmas she could remember. She was able to relax and enjoy herself. And she noticed that all the others had been able to create their own pleasure without her being the self-designated fun-provider.

Here are some suggestions for managing the feelings that surface at this time of year:

- **Decide what you'll need and then make sure you get it.** If you can't be with your family, or all of them, invite friends over to provide company and support. A recently separated woman invited her extended family over for Christmas. As she put it, "I feel the need to have a focus and a reason to decorate the house."

- **Don't dwell on what or who is missing.** Focus on the things you can celebrate (family, health, loving friends, etc.). Absent or departed people needn't be forgotten. A toast and a few thoughtful words are quite appropriate, but shouldn't be prolonged.

- **If you're going to be alone, share your holiday with those in a similar position,** or tell your friends of your situation and ask if you can join them. Don't stand on ceremony or wait for an invitation. "Dropping in" with a small gift at Christmas, an old and welcome custom, is a way of connecting.

- **Share the holiday with people who are having a difficult time** (a friend or neighbor who has suffered a recent loss, is without a job or has no family close by).

- Attend services at your church, synagogue or temple, making connections to both religion and community.

- Volunteer your time to help make the holidays more enjoyable for others. Offering your services to a shelter or community agency can be very rewarding. In my years as a family physician, I was on call every Christmas Eve or Christmas Day so other doctors in our group could be home with their families.

- Don't get drawn into family conflicts. Stand back and become an observer. Watch the family dynamics without making judgments. Avoid family gatherings if you find them too acrimonious or upsetting. Or make a shorter visit.

- Consider going away for the holidays if you feel that staying home will be too painful.

Think about your plans for the holidays. Pull out your calendar and make notes on it.

Consider how you'd like to spend Christmas Eve, Christmas Day, Boxing Day, New Year's Eve, New Year's Day and the adjacent weekends. With whom do you want to share them? Who are the supportive, nurturing people you want to be around? Start placing phone calls to connect with them and to make plans.

Be open and receptive to invitations from others.

Talk about your feelings to people you're close to—or to a trusted professional.

David Posen, M.D.

The little girl who couldn't wait for gift opening has just had her first child. I wonder how Christmas morning will unfold in a few years now that she's the mother!

New Year's Resolutions

Start the Year on the Right Foot

OKAY, THE HOLIDAYS ARE almost over. You got through Christmas, Hanukkah, Kwanzaa and other celebrations. The next big date is New Year's Day. One good thing about January 1 is that it gives us all a fresh start. And none too soon. You've just come through a month in which you probably ate more than you expected, drank more than you intended and spent more than you could afford. Fortunately, the calendar now gives you a chance to make amends and turn over a new leaf for the coming year.

I used to scoff at New Year's resolutions, but a few years ago I actually gave them some thought and jotted down a few things. My motto has always been to keep things simple, so last year I wrote down only three items:

- Leave work at 6:00 p.m.

- Do it now (stop procrastinating).

- Set cruise control at 70 mph/hour (down from 75—in other words,

  drive slower).

I kept the paper handy as a reminder. And even though I strayed a bit through the year, I did pretty well.

It takes twenty-one days to change a behavior.

Here are some thoughts about making New Year's resolutions:

- Make resolutions only if you intend to keep them—not because you think you should.

- Put them in writing. On March 15, 1989, after hearing a speech by best-selling author, Dr. Peter Hanson, I was inspired to write a book of my own. I went home that night, took out a writing pad, and wrote at the top GOAL: To write a book by March 15, 1990." That simple declaration was the start of my first book, *Always Change a Losing Game.* I had been thinking about writing a book for years. But putting it on paper turned the idea into a decision—and a commitment.

- **Limit your number of resolutions.** Some people get ambitious and write down a laundry list of good intentions. Within weeks they feel overwhelmed and give up. A short list of meaningful goals increases your likelihood of success. Three to five items are probably realistic. They can relate to health, relationships, work, money, education, community or spirituality. Just don't overload yourself.

- **Implement your goals sequentially.** Address your resolutions one at a time. Experts tell us it takes twenty-one days to change a behavior. Four years ago, I started doing back exercises using a system of ropes and pulleys. It was a hassle, and I did it only sporadically. Finally, I decided to get serious. Within three weeks, it became a natural part of my morning routine. Pick one item from your list and work on it for a few weeks. When it becomes comfortable, add a second item for three weeks, and so on. You're more likely to succeed and to avoid getting discouraged.

> "The best time to plant a tree is twenty-five years ago. The second best time to plant a tree is now."
> Unknown

- **Be realistic.** Don't make grandiose resolutions and quantum leaps. If you're just getting off the couch to start exercising, don't resolve to work out every day. Commit to a walk three times a week and see how it goes. Then build from there.

- **Be specific.** Don't talk in generalities. "I'm going to cut down on my drinking" should be changed to "I will have a glass of wine with dinner and two drinks on Saturday and Sunday."

- **Be positive.** Rather than saying "I'm going to stop going to bed so late," say "I will start going to bed by 11:00."

- **Express action, not results.** Since you can control only your own behavior, watch how you word your resolutions. Instead of saying "I will get a promotion," say, "I resolve to apply for the manager's job and to upgrade my management skills." The actual granting of a promotion is not in your hands.

- **Go public.** Make your resolutions known to other people. This does not require an announcement on your company bulletin board or a mass mailing to all your acquaintances. Sharing your goals with a few close colleagues, relatives or friends will help make them more real. It also invites their support. If you're reluctant to do this, it might indicate a lack of intention on your part to follow through.

- **Make your resolutions a commitment to yourself.**

Reflect for a few days before you write down your resolutions. Think of the various areas of your life (family, health, career, school, relationships, community, financial). What would you like to improve upon?

Decide on two or three items that are realistic, achievable and meaningful for you.

Word them simply and positively.

Tell your nearest and dearest what you've written. Ask for their support.

Keep your list handy. Review it once a month to monitor your progress.

David Posen, M.D.

New Year's resolutions can help you start the year on the right foot. (Well, actually, you might want to start on January 2, after all those Bowl games are over!)

Wrap-Up
Putting It All Together

W**E'VE COME TO THE END** of our journey through the world of stress. We've talked about work–life balance and how the mind affects the body; caffeine and sleep; anger and worry; procrastination and clutter; technology and deadlines; depression and money; reframing and relaxation; communication and social support; the holiday season and difficult people— and a few other things besides. Through it all, I've tried to demonstrate that there are practical, realistic, achievable ways to deal with stress and that we have more control than we think.

Over my twenty-plus years as a stress counselor and consultant, I've developed a systematic approach for working through any stressful situation. I offer it here as a summary of the ideas in this book. It's based on a simple diagram, and consists of four steps framed as questions.

Let's start with the visual. This is a variation of the Stress Pathway diagram on page 29:

How Stress Happens

Event/Situation (External Stressor)	Lens/Filter (Perception = Reality)	Stress Reaction (Fight or Flight Response)

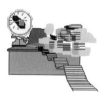 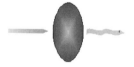 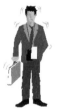

First there is an external event or situation that acts as a trigger (or "stressor"). In other words, something happens. We then process that event intellectually. It's as if we have a lens or filter that makes sense of the event. That filter is our brain, through which our perception becomes our reality. Finally, our body reacts—not to the *event* but to what we *think* about the event, to the meaning we give to it. That reaction is the fight or flight response that we call a stress reaction. And the whole process occurs within seconds.

Here are the first three questions:

1. **How do you know *when* you're having stress?** The first step to dealing with stress is to recognize the signs and symptoms in your body.

2. ***Where* is the stress coming from?** The second step is to identify the source—the problem or situation triggering your upset.

3. ***Why* is this situation upsetting you?** What is it about the situation that's stressing you? What's the self-talk, the interpretations?

The framework for answering these first three questions is summarized below:

How Stress Happens

Event/Situation (External Stressor)	Lens/Filter (Perception = Reality)	Stress Reaction (Fight or Flight Response)

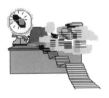 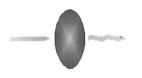 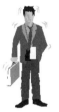

Stressors/Triggers	**Mental Filters**	**Manifestations**
1. Physical/Environmental	1. Interpretations	1. Physical Symptoms
2. Social/Interactive	2. Self-Talk	2. Mental Symptoms
3. Institutional/Bureaucratic	3. Beliefs	3. Emotions/Feelings
4. Major Life Events	4. Expectations	4. Behaviors
5. Daily Hassles		

Once you've become aware of your stress, identified its source and analyzed why it's stressful, the next—and most important—issue is what you can do about it. This leads to the fourth question:

4. *How* **can you reduce the stress?** What strategies and solutions will lower your stress level or help you handle it better?

Just as there are many different *sources* of stress, so too there are multiple options and strategies for *reducing* stress. As a result, I divide the fourth question into three parts:

a) What can you *do* about the situation? (Action Strategies)

b) How else can you *think* about the situation? (Thinking Strategies)

c) How can you *reduce* the actual stress in your body? (Self-Management Strategies)

Some answers to these three questions are given in the three lists in the diagram below. Please note that the lists are not meant to be comprehensive. They're intended only to hit the highlights and indicate the range of choices we have. They also demonstrate that, if one idea doesn't work for you, there are many more you can choose from.

Stress Reduction Strategies

Event/Situation (External Stressor)	→	Lens/Filter (Perception = Reality)	→	Stress Reaction (Fight or Flight Response)

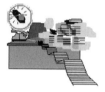   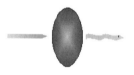   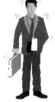

Action	Thinking	Self-Management
1. Physical Change	1. Reframing	1. Exercise
2. Assertiveness	2. Modifying Beliefs	2. Relaxation Techniques
3. Time Management	3. Thought Stopping	3. Time-Outs
4. Problem-Solving	4. Realistic Expectations	4. Sleep ↑, Caffeine ↓
5. Leaving the Situation		5. Social Support
		6. Humor/Play

For *overall* stress mastery, use a combination of all three categories of stress reduction techniques. This is how it all fits together. Here is the organized approach,
with the steps numbered:

Stress Mastery

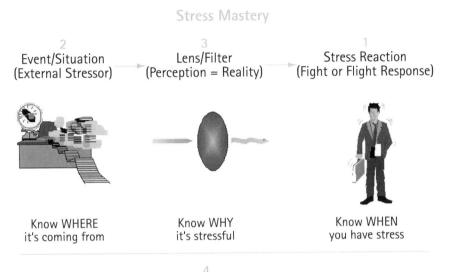

2	3	1
Event/Situation (External Stressor)	Lens/Filter (Perception = Reality)	Stress Reaction (Fight or Flight Response)
Know WHERE it's coming from	Know WHY it's stressful	Know WHEN you have stress

4
Decide HOW you can reduce the stress

4a	4b	4c
Action Strategies (Things you can DO)	Thinking Strategies (Ways you can THINK)	Self-Management Strategies (Take CARE of yourself)

Start to use this system in the weeks and months ahead, and see how you make
out. I assure you, it works!

We're living in a stressful world. There are many things we can't control. But if we
take more control of the things we *do* control, we can keep our stress at an optimal–
or at least a manageable–level. The goal is stress reduction, not stress elimination.
There's no such thing as a stress-free life–and even if there was, it'd probably be
pretty boring. Stress adds spice to our lives and brings out the best in us.

So enjoy the positive stress (*eustress*) that serves you well and reduce the negative
stress (*distress*) that makes you upset and unwell. I wish you the best of luck in your
ongoing journey.

Event/Situation (External Stressor)	→	Lens/Filter (Perception = Reality)	→	Stress Reaction (Fight or Flight Response)

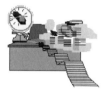 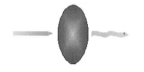 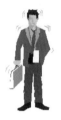

Stressors/Triggers

1. Physical/Environmental
2. Social/Interactive
3. Institutional/Bureaucratic
4. Major Life Events
5. Daily Hassles

Mental Filters

1. Interpretations
2. Self-Talk
3. Beliefs
4. Expectations

Manifestations

1. Physical Symptoms
2. Mental Symptoms
3. Emotions/Feelings
4. Behaviors

Stress Reduction Strategies

Action

1. Physical Change
2. Assertiveness
3. Time Management
4. Problem-Solving
5. Leaving the Situation

Thinking

1. Reframing
2. Modifying Beliefs
3. Thought Stopping
4. Realistic Expectations

Self-Management

1. Exercise
2. Relaxation Techniques
3. Time-Outs
4. Sleep ↑, Caffeine ↓
5. Social Support
6. Humor/Play

Appendix 2: What Is Stress?

WHAT DEFINES A DEMAND?

- The "demand" can be a threat, a challenge or any kind of change that requires the body to adapt.
- The "threat" can be real or imagined.
- The response is automatic, immediate and generalized.
- It is usually perceived as feeling tense, nervous, uptight or anxious.
- The stress reaction is mediated by adrenaline, cortisol and other stress hormones. It is also called "The Fight or Flight Response."

WHAT HAPPENS DURING A STRESS REACTION?

There is an increase in

- Heart rate
- Blood pressure
- Breathing rate
- Muscle tension
- Perspiration
- Mental alertness, and senses are heightened
- Blood flow to the brain, heart and muscles
- Blood sugar, cholesterol, platelets and clotting factors

> "Stress is the non-specific response of the body to any demand made upon it."
> Dr. Hans Selye

There is a decrease in

- Blood flow to the skin
- Blood flow to the digestive tract
- Blood flow to the kidneys

Stress is necessary to life and survival. It can be positive and beneficial (eustress) or it can be negative and detrimental (distress).

Appendix 3:
What Are the Symptoms of Stress?

Symptoms of stress may include any combination of

PHYSICAL SYMPTOMS

- Headache
- Dizziness
- Clenching jaw, grinding teeth, facial twitching
- Chest pain or tightness, palpitations, shortness of breath or air hunger
- Nausea, vomiting, heartburn, indigestion, cramps, diarrhea, constipation
- Shaking, trembling, tremor of hands, clenched fists
- Agitation, restlessness, feeling hyper
- Sleep disturbances (trouble falling asleep, disrupted sleep and/or early wakening)
- Fatigue, weakness, appetite loss
- Loss of interest in sex
- Frequent colds, flu or respiratory infections
- Increases in pre-existing conditions such as migraines, colitis, ulcer, asthma

MENTAL SYMPTOMS

- Decrease in concentration and increased forgetfulness
- Loss of decisiveness
- Decrease in sense of humor
- Mind racing, drawing blanks or confusion

EMOTIONAL SYMPTOMS

- Anxiousness, tenseness or nervousness
- Depression, sadness or unhappiness
- Fear, worry, pessimism
- Irritability, impatience, anger, frustration
- Apathy, indifference, loss of motivation

BEHAVIORAL SYMPTOMS

- Fidgeting, pacing, restlessness
- Compulsive smoking, drinking, overeating
- Nail biting, foot tapping, knee jiggling
- Blaming, yelling, swearing
- Crying, weeping, feeling on the verge of tears

Appendix 4:
External and Internal
Sources of Stress

1. Physical (environmental)

- Noise, crowding, clutter
- Cold, heat, humidity
- Bright lights, low light
- Heights or confined spaces (e.g., airplanes, cubicles, elevators)
- Lack of windows

2. Social (interaction with people)

- Relationship problems (with family, lover, friends)
- Work relationships (with boss, co-workers, customers)
- Crowds, parties, strangers
- Rude, aggressive, critical or competitive people
- Unreliable, moody, indecisive or boring people

3. Institutional (organizational)

(In the workplace, schools, hospitals, government offices)
- Rules, regulations, restrictions, bureaucracy, "red tape"
- Deadlines, schedules, meetings, formalities, office politics

4. Major life events

(Getting married, having a child, moving to a new house or city, death of a spouse or close relative, promotion, loss of job)
- Changes in life circumstances may be positive or negative.
- Stressful impact lasts twelve to twenty-four months, but diminishes over time.
- Effects from different events are cumulative.

5. Daily hassles

(Rush-hour traffic, fear of crime, misplacing things, standing in line, being put on hold, mechanical breakdowns, home maintenance, finding a place to park, rising prices)
- Small, repeated, daily situations can be irritating, annoying and frustrating.

INTERNAL STRESSORS

1. Lifestyle choices
- Health habits: caffeine, insufficient sleep, poor nutrition, tobacco, drugs
- Overloaded schedule, insufficient leisure or poor work–life balance
- Long work hours, shift work, commuting, travel
- Financial overextension
- Social isolation or over-involvement

2. Negative self-talk
- Critical, judgmental, insulting or blaming thoughts, put-downs
- Bossiness ("You should have done ..." and "You must do ...")
- Destructive emotions: guilt, worry, regret, resentment, self-pity, jealousy
- Negative filters: pessimism, cynicism, defeatism, skepticism, suspicion
- Undermining or self-defeating comparisons
- Ruminating, wallowing, overanalyzing and second-guessing

3. Interpretation of events
- Perceiving something as a danger or a threat
- Feeling a lack of control
- Judging something to be a problem
- Jumping to conclusions about other people's motives
- Feeling "not good" about yourself

4. "Mind traps"
- Unrealistic expectations
- Over identifying with roles, job, title, possessions, etc.
- Taking things personally
- Taking on other people's problems as your own
- Exaggerating or generalizing

- Rigidity
- "All or nothing" thinking

5. Belief systems

- Outdated beliefs
- Inaccurate beliefs
- Self-limiting beliefs
- Negative beliefs
- Rigid beliefs

6. Stress-prone personality types

- Workaholics
- Overachievers
- "Type A" personalities
- Perfectionists
- Pleasers
- Caretakers
- Victims

Resources

STRESS

Benson, Herbert, M.D., and Eileen M. Stuart, *The Wellness Book: The Comprehensive Guide to Maintaining Health and Treating Stress-Related Illness* (New York: Simon & Schuster, 1993).

Borysenko, Joan, Ph.D., *Minding the Body, Mending the Mind* (Reading, MA: Addison Wesley, 1987).

Budd, Matthew, M.D., and Larry Rothstein, Ed.D., *You Are What You Say* (New York: Crown Publishers, 2000).

Clarkson, Michael, *Intelligent Fear: How to Make Fear Work for You* (Toronto: Key Porter Books, 2002).

Davis, Martha, Ph.D., Elizabeth Robbins Eshelman and Matthew McKay, PhD., *The Relaxation and Stress Reduction Workbook,* 3rd ed. (Oakland, CA: New Harbinger Publications, 1988).

Ellis, Albert, Ph.D. and Robert A. Harper, Ph.D., *A Guide to Rational Living* (North Hollywood, CA: Wilshire Book Company, 1961).

Hanson, Peter G., M.D., *The Joy of Stress* (Denver: Hanson Stressworks LLC, 2003).

Kabat-Zinn, Jon, Ph.D., *Full Catastrophe Living: Using the Wisdom of Your Body and Mind to Face Stress, Pain, and Illness* (New York: Delacorte Press, 1990).

Posen, David B., M.D., *Always Change a Losing Game!* (Toronto: Key Porter Books, 1994).

Sapolsky, Robert M., *Why Zebras Don't Get Ulcers: A Guide to Stress, Stress-Related Diseases and Coping* (New York: W.H. Freeman & Co.).

Selye, Hans, M.D., *Stress Without Distress* (New York: Signet, 1975).

BURN OUT

Freudenberger, Dr. Herbert J., *Burnout: The High Cost of High Achievement* (New York: Bantam, 1980).

WORK-LIFE BALANCE

Carlson, Richard, Ph.D., and Joseph Bailey, *Slowing Down to the Speed of Life: How to Create a More Peaceful, Simpler Life from the Inside Out* (New York: Harper, 1997).

Edwards, Peggy, Miroslava Lhotsky, M.D., and Judy Turner, Ph.D., *The Juggling Act: The Healthy Boomers Guide to Achieving Balance in Midlife* (Toronto: McClelland & Stewart, 2002).

Hochschild, Arlie Russell, *The Second Shift: Working Parents and the Revolution at Home* (New York: Viking, 1989).

Lazear, Jonathon, *The Man Who Mistook His Job for a Life: A Chronic Overachiever Finds the Way Home* (New York: Crown Publishers, 2001).

Marshall, Dr. Peter, *Two Jobs, No Life: Learning to Balance Work and Home* (Toronto: Key Porter Books, 2001).

Rechtschaffen, Stephan, M.D., *Time Shifting: Creating More Time to Enjoy Your Life* (New York: Doubleday, 1996).

Rossi, Ernest L., Ph.D., *The Twenty-Minute Break* (Los Angeles: Tarcher, 1991).

Schor, Juliet B., *The Overworked American: The Unexpected Decline of Leisure* (New York: Basic Books, 1991).

Smith, Hyrum W., *The 10 Natural Laws of Successful Time and Life Management: Proven Strategies for Increased Productivity and Inner Peace* (New York: Warner Books, 1994).

St. James, Elaine, *Simplify Your Work Life: Ways to Change the Way You Work So You Have More Time to Live* (New York: Hyperion, 2001).

RELAXATION

Benson, Herbert, M.D., *The Relaxation Response* (New York: Avon, 1975).

Kabat-Zinn, Jon, *Wherever You Go, There You Are: Mindfulness Meditation in Everyday Life* (New York: Hyperion, 1994).

SLEEP

Anthony, Camille, and Bill Anthony, *The Art of Napping at Work* (New York: Larson Publications, 1999).

Anthony, William A., *The Art of Napping* (New York: Larson Publications, 1997).

Coren, Stanley, *Sleep Thieves: An Eye-Opening Exploration into the Science and Mysteries of Sleep* (Toronto: Free Press, 1996)

Dement, William C., M.D., Ph.D., *The Promise of Sleep: A Pioneer in Sleep Medicine Explores the Vital Connection Between Health, Happiness, and a Good Night's Sleep* (New York: Delacorte Press, 1999).

Maas, Dr. James B., *Power Sleep: The Revolutionary Program That Prepares Your Mind for Peak Performance* (New York: Villard, 1998).

CAFFEINE

Weinberg, Bennett Alan, and Bonnie K. Bealer, *The World of Caffeine: The Science and Culture of the World's Most Popular Drug* (New York: Routledge, 2002).

TIME MANAGEMENT/PRIORITIZING

Allen, David, *Getting Things Done: The Art of Stress-Free Productivity* (New York: Penguin, 2001).

Covey, Stephen R., *The Seven Habits of Highly Effective People* (New York: Simon & Schuster, 1989).

Covey, Stephen R., A. Roger Merrill and Rebecca R. Merrill, *First Things First* (New York: Simon & Schuster, 1994).

Lakein, Allan, *How to Get Control of Your Time and Your Life* (New York: Signet, 1973).

PROCRASTINATION

Emmett, Rita, *The Procrastinator's Handbook: Mastering the Art of Doing It Now* (Toronto: Anchor Canada, 2001).

Fiore, Neil A., *The Now Habit: A Strategic Program for Overcoming Procrastination and Enjoying Guilt-Free Play* (Los Angeles: Tarcher, 1989).

CLUTTER

Aslett, Don, *Not for Packrats Only: How to Clean Up, Clear Out, and Live Clutter-Free Forever* (New York: Plume, 1991).

Campbell, Jeff, *Clutter Control: Putting Your Home on a Diet* (New York: Dell, 1992).

Culp, Stephanie, *Paper Clutter: Conquering the Paper Pile-Up* (Cincinnati: Writer's Digest Books, 1990).

Hemphill, Barbara, *Taming the Paper Tiger at Home* (Washington D.C.: Kiplinger Books, 2002).

Hemphill, Barbara, T*aming the Paper Tiger at Work* (Washington D.C.: Kiplinger Books, 2002).

TECHNOSTRESS

Shenk, David, *Data Smog: Surviving the Information Glut* (New York: HarperCollins, 1997).

Weil, Michelle M., Ph.D., and Larry D. Rosen, Ph.D., *Technostress: Coping with Technology @ Work, @ Home, @ Play* (New York: Wiley, 1997).

SOCIAL SUPPORT

Ornish, Dean, M.D., *Love and Survival: The Scientific Basis for the Healing Power of Intimacy* (New York: Harper Perennial, 1998).

Pennebaker, Joseph W., *Opening Up: The Healing Power of Expressing Emotions*, revised ed. (New York: Guilford Press, 1997).

MONEY

Dominguez, Joe, and Vicki Robin, *Your Money or Your Life: Transforming Your Relationship with Money and Achieving Financial Independence*, new ed. (New York: Penguin, 1999).

Gignac, Robert M., and Michael J. Townshend, *Rich Is a State of Mind* (Toronto: Wealth Advisory Services, 2003).

Schor, Juliet B., *The Overspent American: Why We Want What We Don't Need* (New York: Basic Books, 1998).

ANGER

McKay, Matthew, Ph.D., Peter D. Rogers, Ph.D., and Judith McKay, R.N., *When Anger Hurts: Quieting the Storm Within* (Oakland, CA: New Harbinger Publications, 1989).

Potter-Efron, Ron, and Pat Potter-Efron, *Letting Go of Anger: The 10 Most Common Anger Styles and What to Do About Them* (Oakland, CA: New Harbinger Publications, 1995).

Williams, Redford, M.D., and Virginia Williams, Ph.D., *Anger Kills: 17 Strategies for Controlling the Hostility That Can Harm Your Health* (New York: Harper Perennial, 1994).

COMMUNICATION

Gray, John, *Men Are from Mars, Women Are from Venus: A Practical Guide for Improving Communication and Getting What You Want in Your Relationships* (New York: HarperCollins, 1992).

Tannen, Deborah, Ph.D., *You Just Don't Understand: Women and Men in Conversation* (New York: Quill, 2001).

DEPRESSION

Greenberger, Dennis, Ph.D., and Christine A. Padesky, Ph.D., *Mind Over Mood: Change How You Feel by Changing the Way You Think* (New York: Guilford Press, 1995).

Rosenthal, Norman E., M.D., *Winter Blues: Seasonal Affective Disorder: What It Is and How to Overcome It* (New York: Guilford Press, 1993).

Solomon, Andrew, *The Noonday Demon: An Atlas of Depression* (New York: Scribner, 2002).

Index

ABC System, 98
abdominal breathing, 163
abusive behavior, 154–56
acceptance, 153
accommodation, 153
action strategies, 190, 191
Adams, Patch, 142
aggressive speech, 143
Always Change a Losing Game (Posen), 77, 140
anger management, 168–71, 202
anticipatory stress, 26
appeasement, 152
appraisal, 151–52
arousal, and performance, 56–57
assertive speech, 143, 156
autonomy, 154, 155
avoidance, 152

balance, 42–44
Bay, Eli, 163
behavior, changing, 185
behavioral symptoms, 20, 194
behavioral therapy, 173
belief systems
    constructive beliefs, 82–83
    general beliefs, 81
    as internal stressor, 198
    power of, 80–81
    work-related beliefs, 81–82
benefits of stress reactions, 17
"Ben Franklin balance sheet," 130–31
Benson, Herbert, 162
the blues, 172–74
boundaries, 55–58, 71
breaks, 84–86
breathing exercise, 163
Brooks, David, 106
Budd, Matthew, 142
buffer time, 72–73
burnout, 42, 90–93, 199
Burn-Out (Freudenberger), 90
buy leisure, 78

caffeine, 65–67
call waiting, 107–8
Cannon, Walter, 35
capacity to deal with stress, 40–41

causes of stress. *See* sources of stress
change, promotion of, 52–54
Chellew, Len, 150
children, and anger management, 168, 171
Christmas. *See also* holiday stress
    emotions during, 182–84
    and illusion of perfection, 180
chronic stress, 19, 36
"closing open circuits," 136–38
closure, 136–38
clutter
    decluttering strategies, 120–21, 122–24
    paper clutter, 122–24
    problems of, 119
    resources, 201
coaching, 176
coffee, 65–67
cognitive therapy, 173
combining your values, 78
comfortable clothing, 73
commitment, 187
communication
    aggravation, 106–8
    content vs. process, 104
    and home chores, 114
    improvement, tips on, 104–5
    language, power of, 142–44
    listening, 105
    resources, 202
    skills, 103–5
    timing, 105
company policy, 51–53
complacency, 134
concern, 134
confidence level, 49
consensus, 52
constructive beliefs, 82–83
control, 155
conversation, art of, 103–5
coping strategies, 157–59
Coren, Stanley, 63, 64
corporate culture, 48–49, 51–54
courage of convictions, 53
Covey, Stephen, 98–99
Creative Worrying, 134–35
criticism, 143
cumulative effects, 24
current circumstances, 33

To contact Dr. Posen for speaking engagements or seminars,
please call or write:

David B. Posen, M.D.
1235 Trafalgar Road
Suite 406
Oakville, Ontario,
Canada L6H 3P1

Telephone: (905) 844-0744
Toll-free: 1-800-806-2307
Fax: (905) 844-4540
E-mail: davidposen@iprimus.ca
Web site: www.davidposen.com